HEALTHCARE REVAMPED:

Empower Yourself Beyond Pills and Politics

Kasia Osuch

Functional Nursing

Functional Publishing
Chicago, Illinois

Details & Contact

Copyright © 2025 by Functional Nursing LLC

Title: Healthcare Revamped: Empower Yourself Beyond Pills and Politics

Functional Publishing LLC
1350 Nottingham Lane
Hoffman Estates, IL 60169
info@functionalpublishing.com

ISBN: 979-8-9926842-0-9 (paperback)
ISBN: 979-8-9926842-1-6 (e-book)
ISBN: 979-8-9926842-2-3 (audiobook)

Library of Congress Control Number: 2025904126

PR Inquiries: Kasia Osuch, kasiaosuch@functionalnursing.com, 847.345.8333
Website: www.functionalnursing.com

Neither the publisher nor the author is engaged in rendering professional advice or services to the individual reader. The ideas, procedures, and suggestions contained in this book are not intended as a substitute for consulting with your physician. All matters regarding your health require medical supervision. Neither the author nor the publisher shall be liable or responsible for any loss or damage allegedly arising from any information or suggestion in this book.

The recipes contained in this book are to be followed exactly as written. The publisher is not responsible for your specific health or allergy needs that may require medical supervision. The publisher is not responsible for any adverse reactions to the recipes contained in this book.

While the author has made every effort to provide accurate telephone numbers, Internet addresses, and other contact information at the time of publication, neither the publisher nor the author assumes any responsibility for errors, or for changes that occur after publication. Further, the publisher does not have any control over and does not assume any responsibility for author or third-party websites or their content.

Dedication:

I dedicate this book to all the caregivers of the world—the young and eager physicians, nurses, and patient care technicians; the experienced ones who feel burnt out and exhausted; the ones feeling depressed, themselves in need of receiving care.

This is for all those suffering secondary trauma; the caregivers who've been injured, and those feeling disappointed, lonely, and defeated. To the frontline emergency staff, paramedics, firemen, and police officers who fear for their own lives as they strive to save others.

This is a shout-out to the respiratory therapists, ultrasound, MRI, and X-ray technicians, unit clerks, and secretaries, whose skills may be less visible to patients and their families but make all the difference in patient outcomes.

To all of those who are not part of the healthcare system directly but who are caring for their loved ones each and every day—please know that you are appreciated. If not for you, where would your loved one have been?

This book is also dedicated to the following coworkers of mine, who died prematurely after living lives of service to others.

NURSE: KINDRA LYNN NELSON

1981 – 2021

An excellent nurse who was a Sexual Assault Nurse Examiner, amongst many other bedside roles, on different units. Kindra will forever be remembered for her dedication and her willingness to help.

She died in her late 30s.

NURSE: MATTHEW T O'BRIEN

1986-2018

Matt had older parents and a brother with disability. His goal was to save up enough money so that he could take care of his brother and his aging parents. He worked nights and would drink Red Bulls to keep himself awake through all the extra shifts he picked up. He will forever be remembered for his smiles, joyfulness, and kindness.

Matt died in his sleep at 32.

NEUROSURGEON: DR. MICHAEL EUGENE STURGILL

1954 – 2019

Dr. Sturgill saved hundreds of lives and for years was the only neurosurgeon working at a level-one trauma hospital. There was no schedule to his life; the hospital had overtaken it. He was always on-call and ready to operate. He was known for his dedication and hard work, and will forever be remembered as a humble and approachable neurosurgeon, who never looked down upon anybody.

Dr. Sturgill ended his life at 65.

NURSE: TRISTIN KATE SMITH

1995-2023

I never worked alongside Tristin, but the letter she left behind after ending her life at 28 years old makes her my very dear soul mate. We share the same abuser, but we must remember that it can't do anything to us if we do not allow it.

I've included Tristin's letter, with its profound message, at the end of Chapter 1.

Preface

Do you feel frustrated with the current healthcare system? Do you find yourself lost within its complexities, unsure of how to make the best decisions for yourself or your loved ones? Perhaps you're a clinician or a bedside care provider, feeling burnt out and trapped in a cycle of exhaustion. Are you weary of the endless cycle of prescribing medications that fix one problem, but create so many new ones?

This book offers a unique opportunity to peer into healthcare through the eyes of a bedside care provider, offering a fresh perspective on the issues we must all confront. It champions a functional approach to medicine that addresses the root cause of disease and enables true healing. It highlights new and innovative ways to function within the system and is full of resources for you to find unity of mind, body, and spirit.

Whether you're a healthcare professional seeking innovative approaches, or an individual eager to prevent or reverse chronic disease through simple lifestyle and dietary changes, *Healthcare Revamped* is written with you in mind. Through self-awareness and lifestyle shifts, it guides you away from disease and towards true healthcare.

Drawing on the work of medical analysts and historians, I explore the complex reasons that underlie the dysfunction of the current U.S. healthcare system. Issues are discussed in a way that will provide you with many *Aha!* moments.

Contrary to what many believe, it is not patient vs. healthcare practitioner. Instead, we are all in this system together, and we must work together to improve it.

About the Author:

Kasia Osuch

Who I am, and Why I Wrote this Book:

After more than a decade as a critical care nurse, I've witnessed firsthand the toll of a healthcare system focused on treating symptoms rather than addressing root causes.

Our healthcare system is in crisis, struggling under the burden of preventable chronic illnesses and overwhelmed caregivers.

Through my own journey of recovery from secondary trauma and burnout, I have come to recognize the transformative power of lifestyle as medicine. I hold a degree in nursing science and board certification in critical care. Determined to spark change, I've pursued advanced training in functional nutrition and nurse coaching, bringing my wealth of experience and expertise to this book.

In this book, I share my insights from the frontline of healthcare, and present my version of 'functional nursing.' It empowers patients through therapeutic partnerships, addresses the underlying causes of disease, and prioritizes prevention as a cornerstone of care.

My message is a call for a **Healthcare Revolution!** One that can curb chronic illness and restore wellness through sustainable, proactive approaches.

Contents

Dedication: 3
Preface 5
About the Author: 6
Acknowledgments 15
Introduction 17

PART 1   25

Chapter 1 - The Healthcare Crisis   27

Poor State of The Healthcare System in the U.S. 28
Issues Leading to Healthcare Challenges 28
Escalating Healthcare Costs 29
Foretold Shortage 30
Wait and See 31
Staffing Shortage 31
Travel and Agency Nurses 32
Low Census Days 33
Floating Nurses 35
Acuity Tools and Appropriate Staff-to-Patient Ratios 37
Exploitation of Nurses 39
Chain of Command 40
McDonald's! 40
Outrageous Salaries 41
Survival Mode: Its Effect on Patients 41
Caring for Caregivers 42
A Letter to My Abuser 45

Chapter 2 - Scientific Medicine 47

Health Education? 48
What Is Scientific Medicine, and How Has It Evolved? 49
The Influence of Money on Science 50
Historical Influence on Healthcare Beliefs 52
Power Dynamics in Healthcare Systems 53
Good Intentions 54
Corporate Philanthropy: Who Pays the Piper? 55
Hospital Funding 56
The Gap Between Rich and Poor 57
Victims of Gun Crime 58
The Challenges of Practicing Scientific Medicine 60
The Complexity of Role Division 60
Illiteracy 61
The Street Laws 61
Teaching vs Primary Care Hospitals 62
Increased Productivity? 63
The Art and Science of Nursing 65
Which Answer is Right? 66
Importance of Real-Life Experience 69
Computerize the Job, Depersonalize the Care 71
Caregiver Shortage, Administration Surplus 71
Unrealistic Goals 72

Chapter 3 - The Sick-Care Model 75

Our Disease-Focused System 76
The Holistic View 77
Quick Fixes 78
Accept, Unite, Include 79
Dividing the Body 80
Specialization in Practice 81
Protocols 81
Increasing Pressure on Nurses 82

Removal of organs: Organectomy 83
Natural Medicine 84
Are Unimportant Organs Important? 85
Treating the Symptoms Rather Than Finding the Cause 87
Death Denial 89
The Death Fighting Dilemma 91
The Time Is Now 93

PART 2 - Reclaiming Health — 97

Chapter 4 - Through Mindfulness to Awareness — 99

Introduction to Mindfulness and Awareness 100
How Mindfulness Connects to Health and Well-being 100
Action and Reaction in Life 100
Responsibility and 'Respond-ability' 101
Importance of Awareness in High-Stress Environments 102
Awareness in Personal Relationships 103
Time Perception and Awareness 104
Mindfulness as a Foundation for Healthy Relationships 105
Practical Ways to Practice Mindfulness 105

Awareness of the System — 106

Dependence on Social Systems 106
Everyone Contributes to The Healthcare System 106
The Reality of Trauma and Healthcare Dependency 106
Transformation of the System 107
Unity of Mind, Body, and Spirit 107
Global Interconnectedness and Environmental Impact 107

Awareness of Personal Bias — 108

Interdependence and Collective Consequences 108
Convenience and Lack of Appreciation 108
Anxiety Caused by Overwhelming Abundance of Choice 108
Information Overload and Manipulation 109

Education and Misinformation 109
Advertisement Revenue Model and Internet Search Engines.......................... 109
Biases in AI Systems 110
Confirmation Bias and Emotional Attachments 110
Awareness is the Key 111

Awareness of Self 111
Acknowledging Unawareness and Bias 111
Perceptions and Biases in Interactions 112
Transforming Relationships Through Awareness.. 112
Liberation from Self-Insertion 112
Reflecting on Personal Behaviors 113

Interoceptive Awareness: 114
Listening to Your Body 114
Role of Interoception in Emotional Awareness 114
Bodily Sensation and Communication.. 114
Interpreting Pain and Sensations 115
Challenges of Ignoring Body Signals 116

Unawareness 116
The Illusion of Health Expertise 116
Symptom Masking and Medication Culture.. 117
Challenges and Solutions 117
Transformation to Health-Oriented Care 118
The Takeaways:... 119

Chapter 5 - Creating Health Inside and Out   121

Simplify 124
Minimize... 128
Recognize 131
Blame Is No Gain 133
Rediscovering Joy 134
The Takeaways:... 136

Chapter 6 - Listening to the Body's Needs — 137

- Conscious Consumers 139
- Applied Science of Nutrition 142
- Fake Food 144
- Food Coma and Coffee Dependence 146
- The Restart Detox 148
- The Fat-Free Diet Disaster 149
- It Isn't the Fat and It's Not the Cholesterol 150
- Inflammation Acute vs Chronic 152
- Understanding Fats 153
- The Whole30 Program 154
- The Keto Diet 155
- The Wahls Paleo Plus Protocol 156
- Lectins 157
- The Mediterranean Diet 158
- The Magic of Cooking 160

What To Eat 163

- Dairy-Free Cheese Sauce Recipe 164
- Homemade Almond Milk Recipe 165
- Making Almond Flour from Almond Pulp 166
- Keto Nut Bread Recipe 167
- Keto Buns Recipe 169
- Healthy Brownie Recipe 171
- The Takeaways: 172

Chapter 7 - Holistic Eating — 173

- What are Nourishing Foods? 174
- Making Healthy Affordable 176
- Preparation 177
- Successful Detoxing 177

Medicinal Soups and Bone Broth 178

- Bone Broth 178

Bone Broth Recipe 180
Chicken Stock and Beef Stock 181
Beef Stock Recipe 183
Vegan and Vegetarian Soups 184
Vegan/Vegetable Broth (Stock) Recipe 185
Vegan Vegetable soup Recipe 186
Tomato Soup Recipe 187
Onion and Leek Soup Recipe 189
Polish Borscht (Beet) Soup 191
Nutrient Dense Polish Barszcz (Borscht) Beet Soup Recipe 191
Beet Kvass 193
Polish Borscht with Beet Kvass 195
The Trash Reward 197
Composting 197
Save Soil 198
The Takeaways: 200

Chapter 8 - From Healthcare to Self-Care   201

Empowered, not Entitled 202
Healing Space 204
Exploring Different Options: 204
Home Birth vs Hospital Birth 204
Embracing Nature 206
My Birthing Experience ....
206
Home Births 207
Birthing Centers 208
Sanitariums & Retreats 208
Spa Alternatives 210
Earthing 212
Mindfulness Practice 213
The Takeaways: 214

Chapter 9 - Eliminating Toxins   215

Toxic Load 216
Harmful Substances in Cosmetics 217
Thickeners, Softeners, Solvents, and Moisture Carriers 218
Simple Ingredients 219
Homemade Natural Substitutes 220
Homemade Multi-Surface Cleaning Spray 221
Homemade Deodorant 223
Easy Coconut Oil Deodorant 224
Super Dry Men's Deodorant 225
Homemade Hand Sanitizer 226
All-natural Facial Moisturizer 227
Homemade Sun Protectors 228
Dr Keesha's Homemade Sunscreen Recipe 229
Homemade Sunscreen with Aloe Vera and Coconut Oil 230
Essential Oils 231
Fungal Infections 231
Tea Tree Oil Ointment 232
Makeup 234
Homemade Blush Recipe...235
Food Products... 236
Pesticides...236
Nothing Fantastic About Too Much Plastic 237
Microplastic 237
Xenoestrogens..238
Bisphenol A (BPA)..238
Phthalates 238
Polychlorinated Biphenyls (PCB's) 239
Plastic Resin Codes, Types, and Common Uses:..........................239
Table:...240
Trash Problem 241
Recycling...242

Wish-cycling 243
"Sacred Economics" 244
Bottled Water 245
Water Filtration Systems 247
Reverse Osmosis Filters 247
Carbon Water Filtration Systems 248
UV Water Filtration Systems 248
Don't Settle for Heavy Metal 249
Natural Ways to Get Rid of Heavy Metals 251
The Takeaways: 252

Chapter 10 - A Functional Approach to Health   253

Why Functional Medicine? 254
What Is Functional Medicine? 255
Functional Nutrition 259
Food Intolerances 259
Acid Reflux 260
Health, Nutrition, and Nurse Coaches 261
Functional Dentistry 262
Homemade Toothpaste Recipe 264
Fluoride 265
Dr. Keesha's Homemade Tooth Whitener 267
Oil Pulling Mixture 268
Functional Orthodontics 269
Lifestyle Medicine 270
Functional Nursing 270
Nurse Coaching 273
Holistic Care 276

Acknowledgments

To **Eric Wyman** for his inquisitive editing, prompt responses, and kindhearted disposition.

To **Carmin C.L. Montante** for her brilliant review and editing of the Cited Sources.

To **Issy Marquez** for her editing and for giving me the courage to pursue publishing.

I would like to extend my heartfelt appreciation to **Catherine Sarah Jarvis** and her husband **Jonathan Jarvis** for their exceptional dedication and unwavering support throughout the creation of this book. Their meticulous reading, insightful feedback, and countless hours of unpaid work have been invaluable to the quality of this manuscript. Catherine and Jonathan exemplify the true spirit of passionate readers and editors, going above and beyond to help shape this book into its best possible form. Their commitment and generosity have made a significant difference, and I am deeply grateful for their contribution.

To **Taylor Dlesk**, my fellow nurse and SICU teammate, for bringing her incredible artistic vision to this book's cover.

Taylor, your ability to blend nursing and art is truly inspiring.

The anatomical heart you created reveals the raw, unembellished truth behind a symbol so familiar to us all—just as the human body, in the hospital setting, is laid bare without glamour or sugarcoating. Yet, beyond its anatomical function, the heart holds something far greater. It captures our essence—our core, the depths of our soul, and our intuition.

The red, continent-shaped patches speak to our profound interconnectedness with the world—a reminder that we are not separate from it but deeply woven into its fabric. They highlight the unity of us within the world and the world within us. The hand cradling the heart embodies strength, ownership, decision-making, and even constraint, reflecting not only the complex nature of our role as nurses and caregivers but also the profound choices each individual must make in relation to the self.

As your nursing "mama," I am so incredibly proud to witness your growth in this profession. Your creativity, compassion, and dedication leave a lasting impact on everyone around you.

Thank you for sharing your gifts with me and with the world.

To **Sadhguru**, for inner engineering and yoga practices, which make anything and everything possible.

To my beloved partner, **Erik,** who put up with my early mornings of 2:00 a.m. to write this book, during our van-life excursions through the world's natural wonders.

To **Rosalba Lopez, Andrea Nakayama, Terry Wahls,** and **Catie Harris** for being my teachers and my mentors, but most importantly for inspiring me to be the practitioners they are, and which I strive to become.

To my **parents, brothers,** and **two sons**. To **Staszek** and **Teresa**, for they have given me the experience of living in their home and the opportunity to experience freedom from having my own.

To **Kinga** and **my nephews**, for reminding me of the joys and challenges of parenthood.

Introduction

"There is a critically ill patient in the stepdown unit who really needs to come here," Anna announced, as soon as I walked into the Surgical Intensive Care Unit (SICU) at the start of my twelve-hour shift. "We've had two Code Yellows overnight, so we were too short-staffed to accommodate the transfer. The patient is a 32-year-old female, who came in with abdominal pain for a few days and a history of gastric sleeve surgery about 3 months ago. Looks septic! I keep going over there and checking up on her. We've intubated and started the Levo drip to increase her blood pressure." Her voice betrayed the urgency.

I put my bag down, took out my light blue stethoscope and hung it around my neck, clipped my badge/key with a small penlight attached to it over the V-neck of my scrub shirt, and checked my right scrub pocket for shears, forceps, pen, and a sharpie. I then checked my left pocket for alcohol wipes and slipped my worn-out nursing shoes on. I was ready.

In the one empty room in our unit where this patient would be transferred, I checked that the ventilator was ready to assist her breathing and that any suction devices needed to clear her airways were also set up and working. The night crew had neatly laid out additional equipment at the bedside table – vacutainers for blood draws, syringes and Micro Pins for medication administration, IV insertion kits, saline flushes, and pulse oximeters to check blood oxygen saturation. The monitor cables were all in place. The room was ready.

I paged the respiratory therapist to facilitate the transfer and rushed over to the step-down unit. At the patient's bedside, the gravity of her condition was palpable. Her blood pressure was dangerously low and barely holding, despite the maxed-out rate on the Levophed drip. Her life was completely dependent on the medication keeping her blood pressure up, and she needed more to make the transfer.

I ran back to my unit and informed the unit resident that the patient required more pressors. I pulled a bag of Vasopressor, another medication to raise blood pressure, from the dispenser while the doctor put the order in the computer. On my way out of the medication room, I started priming the IV tubing to save time.

When I arrived at the patient's bedside, the respiratory therapist was ready for the transfer. I set the newly primed medication in the IV pump and started the infusion; then connected the transport monitor to read all the vital parameters like heart rate, blood pressure, and oxygen saturation. Together, we slowly and carefully moved the patient, including the attached equipment that was keeping her alive, across the hallway and into the SICU.

Once in the SICU, we hung more medication to try to keep the blood pressure from dropping further. Sepsis was obviously the culprit, and knowing the patient's history, her gut must have been the source. Most likely, she had developed an ischemic bowel, where part of the small intestine had died from lack of circulation. She was too unstable to be safely taken to the operating room. We all knew she would not survive another transfer, so Dr. Huang our senior physician that day decided to bring the operating equipment to the bedside and perform surgery in the patient's room. It was her only chance of survival left.

Soon after the decision had been made, a team of operating room nurses, technicians, and residents brought in multiple metal boxes full of sterile equipment to perform the emergency bedside surgery. Dr. Huang and the other SICU resident doctors started preparing the necessary sterile field around the patient's bedside. Everyone was focused and determined to save her life. Adrenaline was pumping through my veins. We were on a mission – all of us working together with one clear goal – to save her life.

After thoroughly preparing the room, the proper equipment, and the sterile field, the surgeons commenced surgery. With a mask over my face and a blue bonnet over my hair, I documented the patient's vital signs at the bedside computer, listening for any call for assistance from the surgeons.

Instead of that call, a shocking statement broke the silence: "It's all dead! All of it is dead."

"What!" I uttered.

"There is nothing we can do," Dr. Huang said solemnly. "We can't save any of it. There is nothing left to save."

"Nothing?" I asked, with genuine disbelief.

"Nothing!" she repeated. "Look, you see how this bowel is purple here, and here and here? That's because it's all dead."

No one said anything. We could all see the purple, lifeless bowel with our own eyes.

Dr. Huang sighed heavily. "All we can do is close it up, speak to the family, and make sure the patient stays comfortable."

As the surgeons closed the patient's skin, a profound silence enveloped the room, punctuated only by murmurs of grief and shock. My head felt heavy with the agony of unacceptance and hopelessness. As I was dealing with my own inner feelings, I could tell everyone else was dealing with theirs.

I continued assisting and documenting, but that moment of inner chaos held me hostage for longer than usual. The impact of this traumatic event will remain with me for the rest of my life.

The silence was all-encompassing, as we each grappled with our own questions and emotions. Was the gastric sleeve surgery the cause of her dead bowel? Did she suffer complications? A blood clot? Why did she need such drastic surgery at just 32 years old? Does she have children? What about her family? How could we prevent such a tragedy in the future? Why is obesity such a growing problem, and are we truly addressing it in the right way, through these invasive procedures?

Immediately after closing the skin and finishing the surgery, Dr. Huang left. The surgical residents were now in charge of segregating the used equipment, while I tidied up the rest of the room. We worked in silence, exchanging only the most necessary technical phrases. We all knew the worst part was yet to come – facing the family.

Witnessing first hand situations like these pain, death, and dying in the ICU – is what has sparked my passion to write this book. Healthcare practitioners in the hospital setting spend a tremendous amount of time, energy, and resources to save one person's life. But what I have realized is that, in most instances, when a patient is in the ICU, the damage to their health has already been done, and the prevention window is often closed.

My long, 12-hour shifts have often left me exhausted, frustrated, and angry. It didn't take me long to understand that the healthcare system in the US is disease-oriented. This approach makes us feel like hamsters stuck on wheels, forever spinning in circles. Instead of focusing on health and prevention, we focus on sickness and disease. We essentially manufacture more illness and disease, while adding layers of financial and environmental strain on ourselves and our planet.

This realization has sparked a desire to bring about change by sharing my experience; there is power in numbers. The more of us who become aware of the dysfunction of our health system, the greater the potential impact will be. However, this is not a concept that many people can easily understand. Even with a healthcare background, the complexity of this issue is enormous. I would like everyone to understand at least the most critical problems we face within this system, because only then can we make educated decisions about the most vital asset we have our health.

Before my nursing career, I knew nothing of the pain people experience when they are fighting for their lives in the ICU; or the difficult decisions their families are forced to make for them. There is nothing easy about dying and, with our scientific advances, the ever-mounting ethical issues have become even more challenging to resolve. Death and dying have become increasingly complicated.

Of course this is not to say that losing a loved one was ever easy, but up until a few decades ago the ability to witness, comfort, and be present with the dying was of paramount importance. Today, however, these are the impossible dreams of a bygone era. Restricted by hospital visitation policies, laws, and regulations, even taking a loved one out of the hospital to die peacefully at home is nowhere near as simple as it once was.

I understand that most of us would rather stay positive and not dare touch upon these sad issues until necessary. However, by not doing so, we are creating a system in which the last moments of our lives are often far from what we would wish for. Dying can be a prolonged process, sometimes lasting weeks, months, or even years. It is often spent unconscious or in agony, without the ability to advocate for ourselves and make decisions. Families may feel trapped within the system, burdened with making the most difficult decisions of their lives regarding the life of another.

Many healthcare professionals, including myself, suffer from burnout and secondary traumatic stress (STS). These are genuinely debilitating syndromes, with each individual affected experiencing and managing them in their own unique way. Although these issues have received more attention in the wake of COVID-19, they have long been significant problems for first responders and for those who care for others. One way I am managing my own professional burnout is by writing this book. The act of writing allows me to share both my experiences and those of many others who feel frustrated and are longing for change.

"Something must be done" is a phrase I constantly hear from my coworkers and other desperate caregivers. For me, this book is that "something" that I am hoping can provoke the necessary change.

Since writing is a form of therapy, please understand that the content of my book comes from a deep well within my soul. My focus is on providing knowledge and education, but I am aware that my personal and professional experiences have influenced my opinions. While reading, I ask that you stay open-minded and recognize that others may have very different perspectives.

The book is divided into two parts. The first part explores my experience in the healthcare system as a clinical practitioner of surgical/trauma ICU nursing, explaining the issues facing our current dysfunctional system. The second part focuses on what each of us can do to live a healthy, fulfilling life. The first part identifies the problems, while the second part offers possible solutions.

Healthcare Revamped is focused on maintaining health and preventing disease. It aims to empower through education and provide actionable steps and concrete guidance for implementing positive changes in our healthcare system.

Part 1

Chapter 1

The Healthcare Crisis

In the United States, medicine came of age during the same period that corporations grew to dominate the larger economy. As corporate capitalism developed, it altered many institutions in society, medicine among them. [1]

Dr. E. Richard Brown

Poor State of The Healthcare System in the U.S.

Healthcare is in crisis.

The United States spends significantly more on healthcare than other developed nations, yet our population's health ranks poorly in comparison with theirs.[2]

Health spending in the U.S. totaled $74.1 billion in 1970, but by 2000, health expenditures had reached $1.4 trillion and, in 2020, the amount spent on health tripled to $4.1 trillion.[3]

According to the Centers for Disease Control and Prevention, more than 117 million Americans, almost half the adult population, live with at least one chronic disease.

Issues Leading to Healthcare Challenges

Besides people having poor health habits, the U.S. healthcare system lacks effective ways to address the root causes of disease or provide care that truly promotes health, well-being, and a high level of quality care. [4]

1 Brown, 2017.
2 Southard et al, 2020.
3 Kurani et al., 2022.
4 Southard et al., 2020.

This is a quote from "Art & Science of Nurse Coaching" by Southard and other authors.

The World Health Organization agrees that the primary reasons identified are lack of engagement and disempowered healthcare consumers, issues that have persisted for many years.

I quote further:

> *"Overprescribing medication has been identified as contributing to serious health problems for the American public. Approximately 80% of the global supply is consumed in the United States, which makes up about 5% of the world population."*

And further on, the report states: *"Medical errors are the third leading cause of death in the United States,"* and that there is a *"lack of continuity and coordination of care."*

Escalating Healthcare Costs

On a per-person basis, health spending has increased sharply in the last five decades, from $353 per person in 1970 to $12,531 in 2020. Adjusted for inflation, this was an increase from $1,875 in 1970 to $12,531 in 2020.[5]

It is fair to say that these are not healthcare but sick-care costs.

Ironically, the term "healthcare" does not accurately match reality. Ours is not a system focused on promoting health; it is a "sick-care" system designed to treat diseases after they have already appeared. Furthermore, in our obsession with treating diseases, we have inadvertently contributed to their proliferation.

---

5   Kurani et al., 2022.

For example, we overly rely on antibiotics to treat bacterial infections. While antibiotics are effective in killing bacteria and treating infections, their widespread, and sometimes unnecessary, use has contributed to the development of antibiotic-resistant bacteria, making infections harder to treat in the long term.

Another example is the focus on managing symptoms of chronic diseases, such as type 2 diabetes, through medications rather than addressing lifestyle factors like diet and exercise. While medications can help control symptoms, they may not address the underlying cause of the disease, leading to its persistence or worsening over time.

The tragic consequences of complications due to bariatric surgery described in the introduction should teach us not to treat obesity in a merely mechanical fashion, but to consider its root causes within the individual. Such causes could be past trauma, low self-esteem, addiction, stress, anxiety, depression, chemical imbalance, genetic mutations, poor diet and lack of knowledge or resources. Surgical intervention may be effective in preventing more weight gain, but it won't resolve underlying problems. Instead, it adds the risk of dangerous complications.

Thus **"sick-care"** is an accurate description of what we now practice in the United States.

Foretold Shortage

The nursing and caregiver shortages which had been discussed and written about for as long as I can remember, have now come to pass. Back in 2009, when I was in nursing school, we were already aware of the statistical data that predicted this becoming a serious issue. We nursing students felt confident that we had picked a good profession since our future jobs would be well-secured.

We were also oblivious to what that meant for us in terms of our workload, unaware of what it is like to work short-handed. We were told that, as the

Baby Boomers grew older, there was going to be an even greater need for nursing care. But now, after the COVID-19 pandemic, the crisis is much more severe than anyone could have predicted.

Wait and See

Back then, we already knew that we would not have enough healthcare professionals to provide adequate care for an aging population. But we failed to act. This approach is the same as our approach to global warming often discussed, but many of the dilemmas remain unresolved. So we wait to see what happens. We wait, thinking that perhaps we'll be fine and all our problems will magically disappear on their own. Just as we wait and see more cataclysms resulting from global warming, we wait to see how the shortage of nurses, physicians and other caregivers will play out.

Well, we don't need to wait any longer. In the same way as more and more ecosystems disappear, while financial interest takes precedence over the stability of our planet, the COVID-19 pandemic brought our already failing system to its knees. Big business, of course, continues to profit.

All over the United States, hospitals are short-staffed to the point where adequate care cannot be provided. Skilled nurses, physicians, and other healthcare providers are overworked, burnt out, and often experiencing compassion fatigue (CF) and secondary traumatic stress (STS), leaving them incapable of practicing their careers. Some feel so hopeless that they have reverted to suicide, which is on the rise among healthcare providers.

Staffing Shortage

The recommended safe nurse-to-patient ratios are constantly being exceeded, and nurses have to take care of more patients than ever before.

During the pandemic, nurses from other units would be brought over to work in the ICUs. They would have to take care of unstable patients on ventilators, having had minimal previous experience, or none at all. Thus, their training took place amid a global healthcare catastrophe. It was so stressful for them that, when called to help, I wasn't sure whom to help first, the patient or the nurse. These conditions pushed many over their limit and many left the workforce, further increasing the shortage of nurses.

But there was never a plan that addressed this eventuality.

Before COVID-19, unit staffing was figured out a few weeks in advance, and many shifts were covered by staff picking up overtime. Since COVID-19, staffing has had to be figured out one day at a time. Nurses are worried that at the end of their 12-hour shifts, they might not be able to go home if there is no replacement. I have often experienced situations in which an entire ICU would be full of sick and unstable patients, where only one or two nurses were on the schedule in place of the five to seven nurses required. Everyone was in a panic and exhausted from working overtime. We were frustrated, disappointed, angry, and at times, in tears, at the same time as caring for and comforting patients and their families. Much of this happens behind closed doors, invisible to patients, their families, and the general public.

Travel and Agency Nurses

The scramble for nurses is often resolved with traveler or agency nurses from outside hospitals, picking up shifts last minute. The full-time staff are too exhausted and too burnt out to work any more overtime, no matter the extra pay. They are trying to hold it together by a thread. Travel or agency nurses come to the rescue. Their 12-week contracts or per diem availability provide some security, and lessen a bit of the stress caused by the lack of staff. Because both travel and agency nurses are usually heavily penalized with fines of up to $500 for any cancellation on their part, regardless of being sick, they make a reliable staff.

Travelers are usually nurses with lots of experience and minimal expectations. They often get the worst assignments since they are contracted and cost the hospital extra money. They are hired to work a specific unit but are often diverted to wherever there is a need. They are usually assigned more patients than the staff nurses. Because of their higher cost to the hospital, upper management justifies this practice by making them 'work for their money.' But this practice fails to recognize that, regardless of pay or cost to the hospital, increased patient-to-nurse ratios are not safe. It is impossible for one nurse to provide adequate care to three or more ICU patients.

Chaos is what travel nurses learn to deal with. Travelers make more money than staff nurses, but they also spend much on out-of-state housing costs. In addition, their contracts sometimes get canceled by the hospital without much notice, leaving them jobless in a state that is not their home, where they most often have contracted rental agreements. If the hospital cancels its contract early without any penalty or reimbursement, it leaves them at a significant loss.

You might be thinking, how is this even legal? Nurse vs. hospital, that's how. CEOs and their associates often rationalize their decision to break these contracts as saving money for the hospital, without any mention of their own multimillion-dollar annual salaries.

In a 2022 piece in Health Affairs Forefront, Vikas Saini, Judith Garber, and Shannon Brownlee from the Lown Institute share their findings:

"As hospital policies and culture have become more aligned with big businesses, hospital executive compensation has swelled…

"… from 2005 to 2015, the average compensation of major nonprofit hospitals CEOs rose by 93 percent, from $1.6 million to $3.1 million, while average hospital worker wages increased by a mere 8 percent in that decade." [6]

Low Census Days

"Low census days" occur when there are fewer patients than expected, and as a result, fewer nurses are needed to provide care on a particular unit

---

6   Saini et al., 2022.

during a shift. In this case, instead of going to work, a nurse may be placed on call. It can be very confusing to learn about the overall nursing shortage within the healthcare system while nurses are being told to stay home and given "low census days." The allocation of nursing staff within a hospital or healthcare facility is a complex process influenced by various factors, including patient census, budget constraints, and workforce management.

Before working in the hospital as a nurse, I had never heard about a low census; it is not something they teach in nursing school. Nor is it something that the general public knows about. I was employed as a full-time ICU staff nurse and was hired to work three 12-hour shifts a week, making 72 hours per paycheck.

I was excited about my first nursing job, until I received a phone call one morning from one of the unit nurses at 5:00 a.m., before the start of my shift. I was given a low-census day, and placed on call instead. I didn't need to come to work at the start of the shift, but I had to be prepared to go in between then and 3:00 p.m. if the need for more nurses arose (for example, if we were to admit several new patients at once). Being placed on call meant that they must be able to reach me by phone, and I had up to one hour to show up for work. Later, I found out that, because low-census days are given away systematically by rotation, whoever hasn't been on call the longest is always next in line. It was my turn since I was new and had never had a low-census day before.

Low-census means that you do not get paid for that day. But because I was waiting to be called, and couldn't take an actual day off, I was compensated at the rate of $2 per hour. This meant that my income was unreliable. If the unit wasn't busy, I would sometimes end up with two low-census days per paycheck. Paying monthly bills was becoming very stressful. I couldn't believe this practice was legal, but when I researched the labor laws, I found that it was indeed legal and that I didn't have any protection. Of course, I could always quit and get a new nursing job, but low-census days occur at just about every hospital.

To make up for the shortfall in my paycheck, I would pick up shifts on other short-staffed units. However, this was resented by other nurses, who were still experiencing their own shortfall in wages. As a result, those low-census days that I was able to make up, they refused to put in the low-census rotation book. This meant that on days when I had a scheduled shift, I would be top of the list for being taken off and put on a low-census day. This ended up with me not working my scheduled workdays, and working during my days off! I then looked for another job at a different hospital to compensate for my lost income, and yet still have time to give towards raising my two sons. These are the reasons why nurses often work more than one job.

The lack of laws to protect nurses, and the rules created in favor of the hospital corporations, exploit those who provide care to the sick. It pushes caregivers into working more than one job, or settling for abusive work environments, which results in high job turnover and burnout. This all adds to the caregiver shortage problem.

Floating Nurses

"Floating" in nursing parlance, has nothing to do with buoyancy. In bedside nursing, "floating" means that instead of giving a nurse a low-census day because there are not enough patients on their usual unit, they are sent to another unit that doesn't have enough nurses that day. This adds extra stress to an already very stressful occupation.

This other unit's layout is unfamiliar, so the patients' room numbers tend to be confusing. Things are done differently in each unit; so while you might know what needs to be done for patients, you don't know how this can be achieved in a different setting. It feels like you are new all over again and this is your first day. Only you get no orientation – no pointers as to what to do. The team that you are used to working with is not there. The staff are new to you, just as you are new to them. There is a different team of physicians that you might not know how to contact. Which one of them should you page? What is their pager number? Much of your time is taken up figuring out where things are and how to document appropriately since that also is very different.

Not knowing the unit makes you feel inefficient and unproductive, even though you often work above and beyond what you are used to since the unit was short-staffed to begin with.

Despite the extra stress, picking up shifts on other units, such as the recovery unit, is precisely what I did to compensate for my low-census days. But I was doing it "voluntarily." I am putting quotation marks around the word voluntarily, since losing income through low-census days was never my choice.

"Floating" is not voluntary; it is assigned. Just as low-census days are recorded, so are floating days. Each time a nurse "floats" to another unit and their name is recorded in the book, whoever was last to "float" is next in line.

Predicting accurate patient ratios in hospitals is impossible, so the idea of floating makes sense. Therefore, nursing positions like float-pull, registry, or agency nurses are hired, knowing that they will be filling in staffing gaps. Since it is more challenging to work in different units which are often the busiest, these nursing positions ought to be rewarded at a higher rate than that of a regular staff nurse.

Unfortunately, hospitals often find alternative ways to avoid these extra costs. The ICU nurses have the most extensive training, so based on their clinical experience, they can be floated to most other units. However, nurses from other departments can't be floated to the ICU without training. Thus, hospitals use ICU nurses to staff other units and as a result, ICU nurses, hired to work on one unit, can be sent off to work at another, sometimes even in the middle of their shift. In these cases, they have to give up their patient assignment for that day and pick up a new one at a separate unit.

In my experience, as with low-census days, float days often create a hostile working environment. Sometimes, nurses would argue about who was next to float, or whether extra shifts worked at other units should be placed in the book and counted as a float day, and how many hours should be taken into account. Nurses would feel furious and frustrated, especially if they had been taking care of the sickest and most unstable patient in the unit, who then dies, and they are no longer required and are told to float. A nursing job is not like factory work, but the insensitivity of this approach by management seems to treat it as such and is a cause of burnout.

Acuity Tools and Appropriate Staff-to-Patient Ratios

In the context of hospitals and staff-patient ratios, "acuity tools" typically refer to methods or systems used to assess the patient's acuity – the level of care required by individual patients. Acuity tools help healthcare providers determine the appropriate staffing levels and allocation of resources based on the severity of patients' conditions.

Well-equipped hospitals, for example those awarded Magnet Status, which is given by the American Nurses Credentialing Center (ANCC) for meeting specific criteria of excellence in nursing and patient care, use specific software to help them allocate resources and staff based on the constantly changing needs of the patients.

Unfortunately, many hospitals still use the less effective number grid. In such a system the focus is placed on the number of patients regarding the amount of nursing staff, rather than considering the patient's acuity level. Management's concern is whether the ratio of nurses to patients matches their approved grid. As long as the numbers match, all concerns raised by the staff nurses are dismissed. However, appropriate staffing in a hospital setting should never be reduced to numbers. Each patient's acuity level is pivotal in determining safe and appropriate staffing.

Should a patient be critically unstable, requiring constant attention and intervention, then they are designated 1:1 meaning that one nurse is assigned to take sole care of one patient.

What the grid system fails to address is that in such instances a whole team is required. Not one nurse, but two, three, or even four nurses, plus medical students and unit residents must work together to save that one life. While one hangs medications and documents vital signs, the second fetches appropriate equipment, the third sets it up or might need to run to the blood bank, and the fourth might be busy on the phone coordinating an emergent plan of care with other physicians and the rest of the team.

Another example of how numbers misrepresent the true situation on a unit would be the diagnostic tests and procedures done outside the units, commonly called trips. In these cases, ICU patients must always be accompanied by a nurse; if they are intubated and on a ventilator, they must always be accompanied by a nurse and a respiratory therapist.

I could be assigned to have two patients, but be gone from the unit for much of my shift. One of my assigned patients may need multiple trips to get an MRI and a CT scan, while the other gets a video swallow study or a VQ (lung function) scan. Multiple patients may require multiple trips out of the unit, which leaves a shortage of nurses with a surplus of patients. In addition, a nurse might get caught up assisting with a bedside procedure like a bronchoscopy or central line placement. Who takes care of their other patients?

Trips and bedside procedures, including emergencies like resuscitation, immediately change staff-to-patient ratios. In situations like these, mere numbers do not reflect the intricate details of nursing and patient care.

A better way of determining safe ratios is for well-organized, effective acuity tools to be used. Unfortunately, many hospitals still do not use them but persist with a numbers-based approach.

Exploitation of Nurses

As Brown says,[7] the state's emphasis on technological medicine has "ignored some of the most important determinants of disease and death." Economic and political forces maintain control over the medical market. This private market "is a contradiction that now plagues the state and the corporate class as the demand for national health insurance grows."

As a country we strive to increase our economic development, hoping it will provide equal opportunities for all our citizens. Ironically, our economic development owes much of its success to the exploitative measures exerted on the working-class.

Hospitals, in line with other big corporations, exploit their workers. An example of such sharp business practice: If a nurse calls in sick, their first two days off are treated as vacation days, instead of being taken out of their sick bank hours. Their vacation days, or paid time off (PTO), are based on the hours worked. This paid time off must be paid even if it is not used; for example, when the job terminates. Sick time is also provided for, but can't be cashed out like vacation time. Sick time hours, if not used, are lost at the time of job termination.

The hospital would rather have their caregiver employees lose their vacation time, rather than give them a much-deserved sick day. This practice was so outrageous that it was later chnaged.

Another example of exploitation would be the low census days mentioned previously. Nurses are given the option to pull money from their vacation budget to substitute for income lost due to a low census day. How is it fair, or legal, to hire a full-time employee and promise them appropriate compensation, including vacation benefits based on their employment status, when it is all subjected to the constantly changing number of patients? In reality, none of these benefits are guaranteed.

---

[7] Brown, 2017.

Chain of Command

As with employees of any other corporation, nurses are instructed to take any issues they have up the chain of command. There should be a well-defined protocol to resolve problems effectively; but in reality, the chain has gotten so long and stretched out that, should one be lucky enough to reach any influential personnel, it seems as if the two sides are speaking a different language. The gap between the business side of running a hospital and running floors and taking care of patients has grown out of proportion.

My effort in writing this book is to raise greater awareness concerning the disconnect between bedside staff, patient needs, and the CEOs and their business associates. When nurses advocate for patient safety, their pleas are often ignored. Sometimes, when threatened by the labor unions, the administration will promise a change. It will improve staffing until the threat lessens, only to revert later to the same dysfunctional practice.

McDonald's!

How surreal the situation has become was brought home to me at a meeting between management and bedside nurses. In order to explain its financial strategy of checks and balances, the management representative compared our hospital to McDonald's – this was while attempting to persuade us to sign a change to the nurse/patient grid that was of no benefit to patients or staff. Nurses were outraged by this comparison. We wanted, at this meeting, to advocate for safer staffing; for ensuring the safety of patients who would die without proper care, and who can't advocate for themselves only for our lives' work to be compared to a burger-production business.

I'm sure it's much easier to do checks and balances when you think of patients as numbers or in this case burgers but it doesn't feel like that to us. Dedicated nurses often compromise their well-being to help patients, taking on extra shifts, not for the money, but to prevent their patients and coworkers from being left short.

Outrageous Salaries

The CEOs' outrageously high salaries compared to bedside care providers are appalling. According to the Economic Research Institute (ERI):

"In 2018 Bernard Tyson, then-CEO of nonprofit healthcare giant Kaiser Permanente, made nearly $18 million, making him the highest-paid nonprofit CEO in the nation. The previous year, the top ten highest-paid nonprofit health system executives each made $7 million or more." [8]

Nurses are constantly being pressured, manipulated, and coerced into taking on more responsibilities, patients, and shifts to help take care of an increasingly sick population. Cuts to pay, expensive insurance, poor benefits, and inadequate retirement plans are always attributed to the hospital's "lack of money." There is no mention of the ever-increasing amount of managerial positions (these also cost money), diverting resources away from patient care to maintain the bureaucratic structure.

Following the COVID-19 pandemic, a shortage of nurses, resulting in an increased demand, has seen nursing pay increase – rightly so, in my opinion, considering the increased level of stress the crisis caused. Now, there is an active effort being made by the legislation to cap nursing pay. Why is no effort being made to limit the CEOs' multimillion-dollar annual salaries or their million-dollar bonuses? Why, instead of cutting staff, having low census days, canceling traveler nursing contracts, and the like, don't *they* take a pay cut to save the hospital money? Their loss would hardly equate to that of those who provide care at the bedside.

Survival Mode: Its Effect on Patients

Following the pandemic, hospitals lost a lot of full-time nursing staff. These gaps are being filled by contracted travel, agency, and per-diem nurses. Another of the pandemic's effects on the profession sees nursing graduates unable to obtain previously mandated clinical hours as part of

---

[8] Saini et al., 2022.

their training. On becoming full-time nurses, they now need to be given this training by experienced nurses to ensure safe practice. Previously, these deficiencies would be remedied by experienced preceptors; but currently, there are simply not enough experienced staff to do this.

It is now a fact that new graduate nurses are being taught by traveler or agency nurses since they are often the ones staffing the hospital units. At times, they can be the only ones working the unit, and there is not a single staff nurse employed by the hospital.

This practice is detrimental to the quality of patient care. Even though the contracted nurses are knowledgeable and have plenty of experience, they are new to the hospitals and not as familiar with specific hospital protocols or resources as full-time staff nurses would be. They would not be orienting new nurses in normal circumstances—they often need a resource nurse themselves!

Still, all the previous laws and regulations to ensure patient safety are being disregarded, due to the nursing shortage. Survival of the fittest is now the law within our hospitals. But by talking in these terms, whose survival do we mean?

Caring for Caregivers

Every nursing plea about safe staffing, better equipment, more supplies, and improved working conditions is the result of our concern for our patients. Our pleas are not for ourselves. They are on behalf of those we represent. For us, it's all about the patients.

But from the hospitals' point of view, the health and safety of caregivers should be as important as the health and safety of those they serve. Safe spaces should be provided for nurses to relax and take naps at break time, between their shifts, or at the end of night shifts before driving back home. Nurses, exhausted from working twelve or even sixteen-hour shifts, and worried about getting fired, should not have to hide in cars or empty conference rooms to catch up on sleep.

It is time to realize, belatedly, that caregivers also require care. No matter how technologically advanced a hospital might be, health care cannot exist without nurses.

We need to feel supported. Skilled nurses are of tremendous value to our patients and to society, but their skills lead to them being exploited. It may even be that they have no choice but to resign. Burnout and secondary traumatic stress (STS) among caregivers is a real, not imaginary, issue. So that we can better help our patients, we also need help.

During the COVID-19 pandemic, nurses were given lunches and dinners by the local communities and their restaurants. The delicious food would often come with beautiful inspirational messages, expressing how loved and appreciated we all were for our hard work. I have rarely experienced anything so moving. During that time, we were never hungry - at least, not because of lack of food. If we were, it was because of a lack of time.

Many caregivers felt supported and uplifted by the "Nurses are Heroes!" messages that appeared at store-front entrances and all around our communities. But for some of us, overwhelmed with feelings of grief, helplessness, anger, and frustration, they highlighted our disappointment in a healthcare system that was failing – despite years of predicted caregiver shortage.

During that time, there was little about nursing that felt close to heroic the piercing screams of our patients' loved ones grieving their sudden death the images of our patients' swollen bodies with open blisters and peeling skin, brutally carved into our memories facial expressions of excruciating pain caused by each and every turn that, to this day, continue to haunt us in our dreams. Desperate for miracles, we turned them face-down to a prone position[9] to improve their dropping oxygenation. Helplessly, we administered life-prolonging medications to the dying.

---

9 Prone position means lying face down or flat on your stomach. Turning an unconscious and unstable ICU patient who must stay connected to life-supportive measures like the ventilator and multiple IV medications at all times is not simple and in regular circumstances requires a specific type of a turning bad. During COVID there weren't enough of these beds to fit the needs of our patients, so a new protocol of how to safely turn patients without specialized equipment was developed. It takes an entire team of trained nurses to safely turn one ICU patient face down into a prone position.

HEALTHCARE REVAMPED

So, as I ate the delicious food sent to our unit, tasting the different cuisines and receiving the beautiful messages attached, my heart was filled with both profound gratitude and sincere sadness. I wondered if the people of our community, so capable in organizing and delivering such caring gifts to us, would believe to what extent we nurses were being exploited by the system.

The same sadness and disappointment in our system was expressed so painfully by Tristen Kate Smith (a 28-year-old ER nurse whose name I've mentioned in the dedications) in this letter to "her abuser."

Here is her letter:

A Letter to My Abuser[10]

Ever since I was young, I expressed interest in healthcare and becoming a nurse, so I began my study. I gave my heart, my body, and my mind to you; dedicated long hours and days and gave you my all. I have cried with patients, with their families, and for them. I held their hands, and they held mine as I moved forward in my nursing career. My patients and their families have been there for me, supported me, and reminded me why I do what I do. I thought that was enough; this would be all I needed to carry me through my career. I told you I would be there through the good and the bad, but you have taken my heart and slowly crushed the goodness it had. You love-bombed me with affection, and you told me I was going into a career that matters. I could make a difference.

You made me feel comfortable, despite the rumors of your abusive past rumors I didn't want to believe. The compliments, the pizzas, and the thank you letters gradually had less meaning to me, though. The staff I worked beside began to go away. In your eyes, these staff were "unnecessary," but it came at a high cost for the advertised "quality care" provided to our patients by those of us who were left.

You asked my colleagues and me what we needed to help patients and improve satisfaction scores, and we told you the truth. But then you sent us to online courses that taught us to just smile more and be friendlier to the patients. That's when I began to understand your true cruelty and manipulation.

I remember the first time I heard about nurses getting hit. I remember that you asked them what they'd done or didn't do to prevent it from happening. "Don't protect yourself by fighting back," you said, "just lay with your hands over your head and wait until security comes." You created an environment of fear and blame in a place we already felt unsafe.

---

10   *The Oakwood Register,* 2024 (accessed online; see bibliography for full details).

HEALTHCARE REVAMPED

You blamed us for things out of our control. You criminally charged my colleagues for things that happened as a direct result of your own actions. The law doesn't protect us, and neither do you.

I no longer feel like you care about me or the people you say you serve. I sit at my front desk just waiting for someone to walk in off the street and shoot my patients and me: you do not care about keeping us protected. You haven't provided even the slightest amount of security to keep us safe. You use and exploit us to line your pockets, using the common citizen's money for overpriced healthcare.

You are a narcissist. I can see you for what you really are. You say you care, but you ignore us while we beg on our hands and knees. You tell us we do so much and that we put up with so much. But when we dare to think we are finally going to get the love and support we deserve, we get a pizza party and free pens for the "healthcare heroes."

I so desperately want to continue to help people, but I cannot stay in this abusive relationship.

Each day, you ask me to do more with less.

You beat me to the point that my body and mind are black, bruised, and bleeding out.

I'm only sorry to my patients and colleagues. You deserve so much better, but my abusive partner is relentless.

If I stay, I will lose my sanity and possibly my life forever.

Chapter 2

Scientific Medicine

Instead of medicine liberating us from the suffering and dependency of illness, we find that its oppressive elements have grown at least as rapidly as its technical achievements.[11]

Dr. E. Richard Brown

Health Education?

To understand scientific medicine, let's go back to our first years in school. Let's remember how we were taught about the world around us. Most of our education did not come from direct experience; rather, we learned by listening, reading, and watching videos. Sheltered from all the elements, we learned about wind, water, earth, and fire. Sitting for 8 hours a day in a classroom, from as early as five years old, we have learned about the world outside. Then, at the age of puberty, in a "health" class, we were told about hormones, the reproductive system, and sex, although up to this point, many of us had studied no human biology. With no reference to the stomach, heart, lungs, brain, liver, spleen, gallbladder, kidneys, thyroid, etc, we learned about penises and vaginas, as if they make up most of our human body. Perhaps our teachers couldn't skip those two, even if they wanted to.

Later, after more years of exams and studying, we were then led to believe that rather than the penis or vagina being our most important organ, we should give a standing ovation to the brain.

For those like me, who wished to explore beyond our "health" class education and become nurses, doctors, physical, occupational, or speech therapists (amongst many other professions), we were required to gain extensive knowledge of human anatomy and physiology.

---

11   Brown, 2017.

As we had been taught previously at school, knowledge was imparted to us in a package (as if in a zip file). By now, we had become proficient at absorbing information in a pre-digested form. Living off Ramen noodles for breakfast, lunch, and dinner, so as to afford the school loans, we were finally able to fill in the gaps left by previous "health education" classes. Compromising all our bodies' normal functions along the way sleep-deprived, overweight, and broke we somehow managed to survive and make it to our graduation. With all our hard-earned knowledge packed inside our brains, we were considered ready to practice.

Without any experience of how it feels to be well-rested, nourished, and stress-free, we began our careers in educating others on how to be healthy.

What Is Scientific Medicine, and How Has It Evolved?

Health, and staying healthy, is not that complicated, so where did we go wrong? I would often wonder about this at work while attending to the sick. It doesn't take a doctor with four years of pre-med, four years of medical school, and additional years of residency and fellowship, to teach their patients about a healthy lifestyle. Everyone should be taught, for instance, that high-fructose corn syrup is added to most products sold at the grocery store; and they should also be taught of the harm it causes and the health issues that result. This fact should be universal knowledge, so that people would not wish to consume it. Yet I learned nothing of it in nursing school.

My Bachelor Degree in nursing contained no course on nutrition. Doctors graduate after seven or more years of college with one semester of nutrition at best. No wonder some gastroenterologists I've talked to deny any impact of diet on their patients' health. We focus on learning the complex science of the human body, yet overlook the basic, but crucial, factors of lifestyle, food and nutrition, which have the greatest influence on our health.

Why aren't greater efforts being made to inform the public of the crucial part lifestyle plays in our health? Because our focus has been elsewhere.

Scientific medicine focuses on evidence-based practices and systematic approaches to diagnosis and treatment. It applies principles used in the world of industry to "scientifically manage" health care.[12] Within healthcare, we see increased standardization, specialization, "time and motion studies" – to improve efficiency, "control and supervision" – giving managers oversight to ensure standards have been adhered to, and "profit maximization" to ensure that the workforce acts in line with this business model. Healthcare became a powerful and lucrative enterprise, with more people to diagnose and treat than we could have ever imagined.

Scientific medicine represents our technical and scientific capability, which allows for more advanced disease treatments, but disregards healthy lifestyle and prevention. Surely this limits its usefulness. We have increased our ability to treat disease while producing more diseased people than ever before.

The Influence of Money on Science

This fixation on science and technology has long been a diverting tactic within the healthcare and pharmaceutical industry. Doctors are incentivized to treat existing illnesses, often through interventions requiring medications or procedures, rather than preventing them. This results in a reactive healthcare system focused on "sick care" rather than proactive health promotion. While we have all benefited from the incredible results of scientific advances – minimally invasive robotic and laparoscopic surgeries, for example – we have lost sight of the benefits of traditional medicine.

Have you ever wondered why your doctor never mentions alternative options rather than using prescription medications for your condition? Why they don't mention a specific diet to lower the inflammation in your body? Why do they ignore supplements, acupuncture, or other forms of relaxation and stress reduction? Why are herbs or homeopathic medicine never mentioned?

---

12   O'Neill Hayes et al., 2021.

Not only does none of this receive attention, but any non-medical treatment is often disregarded or ridiculed. That's because it is not "scientific medicine."

What about functional (sometimes known as holistic or restorative) medicine? What about medical practices that enable the body to heal itself, instead of merely treating symptoms? What about the most obvious and most commonly performed act of sustaining life, which is through sleep, food, and nutrition?

I will go into much greater detail about functional medicine in the second part of the book; for now, let's acknowledge that in conventional medicine, no treatment is regarded as valid if it hasn't been scientifically studied.

Healthcare practitioners are taught to only use evidence-based practice. While I agree with practicing based on the evidence, I am not ignorant of the fact that scientific studies are being financed and publicized only if they are profitable. In spite of an ever-increasing amount of evidence that suggests food additives are harmful, scientific studies on this subject remain few and far between. Why is this? Additives provide the food industry with increased profits; therefore, much financial support is directed toward silencing this evidence and manipulating the data. Studies that would benefit the general public in the most straightforward ways, but do not bring profit to wealthy sponsors, are being left undone. It is easy for the medical profession to disregard this omission.

Doctors are often unaware that their bias against, and ignorance of, alternative ways to cure disease results from the profit-based system that is American healthcare today. They don't realize that their education, which informs their medical practice, has been designed by significant political forces that they are helping to propel.

Historical Influence on Healthcare Beliefs

The notion that disease itself, rather than poverty or other social problems, is the root of all unhappiness is an example of such influence.

In his book: *Rockefeller Medicine Men: Medicine and Capitalism in America*, (2017), the founder and director of the UCLA Center for Health Policy Research and a professor at the UCLA School of Public Health, E. Richard Brown, reviles what was proclaimed by Frederic Gates, an individual who, as guardian of Rockefeller's investments, had a large influence on American life.

Gates' doctrine was that disease, not poverty, was the supreme ill of human life. Paraphrasing Gates, Richard Brown explains these pernicious ideas:

It is clear whence comes the unhappiness. It comes not from the unequal distribution of wealth, sickening working and living conditions, miserable and alienating work, tension caused by frequent and prolonged unemployment, economic insecurity, and competition among those whose sights are set on higher stations in life... It is not poverty or one's place in the capitalist class structure that breeds misery; it is a disease that is a technical, not a social problem.[13]

Further on, he writes:

"Rockefeller money did not support medical research that intestates the relationship of social factors to health and disease. In its first decade, the Rockefeller Institute focused its resources on chemistry, biology, pathology, bacteriology, physiology, pharmacology, and

---

13   Brown, 2017.

> *experimental surgery. It ignored the impact of the social, economic, and physical environment on disease and health."*[14]

The oil magnate John Davidson Rockefeller Sr., and his trusted advisor, the Baptist pastor Frederic Taylor Gates, were two of the most influential men in the development of American capitalism and the modern healthcare system. Although great philanthropists, their denial of poverty and other socio-economic influences on health still blights current healthcare practice.

Power Dynamics in Healthcare Systems

It may be hard to imagine that our current systems, which profoundly influence our lives, were primarily developed by just a few wealthy and, therefore, influential individuals.

Because of their wealth, these individuals had the power to express their beliefs and implement their ideas. Often, circumstances aligned to place them in positions of influence, which they originally couldn't have imagined. Rockefeller was not born into wealth. His accumulation of wealth started with steel, essential for building the railroads used to move troops and supplies for the Union Armies during the Civil War. Helped by the war, Rockefeller's profit proliferated, allowing him to invest in the oil industry, and making him one of the wealthiest and most influential men in US history.

Gates would help manage Rockefeller's wealth. Together, based on their beliefs, but also in line with their interests, they built philanthropic capitalism. Money was gifted only when it would be returned with interest. Together with other wealthy and privileged individuals, they have built the system we are experiencing today. We benefit from its advancements while also suffering from its problems.

---

14   Brown, 2017.

Instead of spreading health and well-being to others, power is still exercised to create more wealth for those who already have it. That is not to say that money and power can't be used in more appropriate ways, but the reality is that high-tech solutions are often expensive and inaccessible to marginalized populations, exacerbating inequalities. The current healthcare system is failing us miserably, a direct consequence of the widespread misuse of money, power, and resources.

It is nigh on impossible to stop this domino effect of actions and consequences. However, it is my hope that, unlike the dominoes, we may be able to accomplish our goal without all the pieces falling.

Good Intentions

I am not saying that scientific medicine has not yielded fantastic results and major breakthroughs in our understanding and practice of medicine. But, at the same time as its ever-increasing technical requirements have given rise to more and more career paths for physicians, medical scientists, researchers and professors, there has also arisen an elite who have a material interest in promoting it.

The pursuit of scientific medicine was begun with good intentions. Scientific medical education was seen as the best way to learn and practice medicine. However, over time, it both dominated and limited our focus on providing care. It has played a major role in creating the challenges we all see around us today.

Good intentions are not enough to produce a good outcome. We must now acknowledge that good intentions do not always end well with regard to the healthcare system today. In healthcare, scientific medicine was intended to cure all diseases, but as a result, it has produced a predominantly unhealthy population.

Let me give an example: Parents love and care dearly about their children. They always intend the best for them. No parent likes to hear their child crying, and therefore they do whatever they can to make the child's sadness go away. But, despite the best intentions, their actions might encourage the crying, or worse, escalate it to a full-blown temper tantrum. Intention does not always determine the outcome. It is nigh on impossible as a parent to always get things right, but I believe that the practice of awareness, as I explain in Chapter 4, can help us in reacting to these and other situations with a better result.

Self-awareness allows us to choose a course of action with a better understanding of its impact. Just like the parent with a crying child, none of the doctors or nurses I have ever worked with wanted to hurt their patients. They all wanted to help.

Back in the day, when as teenagers we were choosing our profession, none of us were aware of the system that we were to become a part of. At that idealistic age, what we wanted was to fix a broken world. With good intentions and an idealistic outlook on life, we became doctors, nurses, teachers, engineers, and social workers. Putting our faith in education, we worked hard to make our dreams a reality.

Now, it is disappointing to realize that fixing the world is more complicated and a lot harder to accomplish than we once thought, and that perhaps it is not the world that needs fixing, but rather ourselves. We should realize that our hard-earned knowledge derives from a manipulated education system.

Corporate Philanthropy: Who Pays the Piper?

Where has the money come from to finance all these scientific medical schools? Surely, those who provided the capital will call the tune.

Rockefeller's wealth had a far-reaching influence on our present-day healthcare system. Both he and his assistant, Fredric Gates, used the money to hold on to their power through the influence of charitable giving – i.e. corporate philanthropy. They gifted institutions to create the system they wanted and benefited from. A century later, the system still stands strong today.

None of these great philanthropists had evil intentions. They did what a lot of us do; they tried to help as they saw fit. The fact that they had much greater means than the rest of us allowed them to make a far greater impact on our country. However, their use of donations, although well-intentioned, served to reinforce their own status and secure their own wealth and privilege. This further reinforced the gap between rich and poor.

Their intentions might have been good, but the consequence of their actions proves otherwise to this day.

Even if science identifies the causes of diseases, and technology develops cures, medical care cannot improve public health or reduce suffering if people cannot afford it.

Hospital Funding

Hospital funding is not easy to understand, nor is it transparent. We have private insurance, Medicare, and Medicaid. Things get even more complex when considering safety net hospitals. In addition, many hospitals depend on corporate philanthropy, where businesses and corporations make charitable contributions towards social and community causes, including hospitals. Hospitals receive such donations to fund medical research, to purchase equipment, and to support patient-care programs.

On the face of it, it seems admirable for a corporation to donate millions of dollars to a good cause: for example, to help sustain a safety-net hospital in need, or to provide it with new technological equipment. But in reality, it may be politically motivated. Companies often receive tax breaks for their charitable donations, which means that taxpayers are effectively subsidizing the political agendas of special interest groups through these tax incentives. [15]

Nor do these donations resolve the root cause of why a particular hospital requires repeated injections of cash to patch up failures and prevent it from closing. It is like putting a band-aid over a dirty wound. Wouldn't you

---

15   Wallheimer, 2018.

want to clean it first, and see what's going on, before you patch it up? By patching without exploring the cause, the wound could become infected even life-threatening.

These "patch-up" donations disguise a more significant problem. The "mercy" behind these donations highlights the gap between rich and poor, and the fundamental issues of segregation. It makes a failing system continue. It makes a safety net hospital that serves impoverished communities dependent on people with privilege and power. Instead of reinforcing such dependence, the effort should be placed in empowering the people of these communities; to let them take charge and become skilled at making the best decisions for themselves and their community, including local hospitals.

The Gap Between Rich and Poor

A coworker turned to me one day during the change of shift and asked, "Kasia, do you know what is the biggest determinant of one's health in the U.S.?"

Curious, I replied, "What is it?"

She answered, "It's the ZIP code!"

As she began to explain an article she had read, it all made sense to me. The ZIP code determines everything. From the quality of one's education, including extracurricular activities, to neighborhood safety, and exposure to violence, all the way to healthcare and nutrition, including access to fresh fruits and vegetables – all are predetermined by one's ZIP code.

I drive 36 miles to work. Not because there aren't any hospitals nearby, but because I choose to work at a safety net hospital that provides healthcare to individuals, regardless of their insurance status or ability to pay.

Thirty-six miles is a short distance compared to the leap in surroundings. It almost feels like space travel and I have landed on a different planet. In that short distance, I seemingly travel back in time as well. I started out driving through neighborhoods of single-family homes, each front yard neatly landscaped, where the grass is kept shortly trimmed in summer months, and holiday lights changed each season. I pass many grocery stores and supermarkets such as Jewel, Mariano's, Amazon Fresh, and Whole Foods; I pass many schools, playgrounds, forest preserves with lakes, and even an outdoor gym. I see joggers at 5 a.m., getting their early morning workout.

Once on the highway, I leave these neighborhoods behind and a new reality hits me. At the first light, I see a homeless man begging for cash. He used to sell newspapers just a few years ago, but with the arrival of the internet and cell phones, had to switch to little bags of popcorn. I guess the popcorn didn't sell any better than the newspapers.

The street is narrow, and the sidewalks are full of scattered trash from fast-food containers, like soda cups and paper bags. The multi-story housing apartments are intertwined with smaller buildings, so close together there is no space for any grass to grow concrete everywhere. I pass abandoned buildings with plywood or cardboard covering the windows, and instead of holiday decorations, I see the obnoxious blue light of the street cameras.

Gone are the joggers, to be replaced by pedestrians, some drunk or high, unable to walk in a straight line. I see sleepers on the bench of the bus stop, some talking to themselves acting crazy, others limping due to their disability while smoking cigarettes. I don't pass a single supermarket or a grocery store, only a fast-food hot-dog joint a food truck where people wait outside in line.

I make sure my gas tank stays full enough to get me back home, and always drive the main streets so that I stay safe.

Victims of Gun Crime

Whenever I have been working in one of the hospitals near my home, I've never had to treat a patient for gunshot wounds. Here, just 36 miles southwest, in the surgical intensive care unit (SICU), caring for violent crime victims is mostly what we do. The hospital serves mostly Black and Latino patients and, judging by the nature of their injuries, it is a war zone. We are not a pediatric unit, so 15 is the youngest we see; most patients are between 16 and 50 years of age.

We don't have the fancy equipment and sophisticated computer programs the other hospitals might have, but we serve patients with critical wounds and injuries that others don't see. Some patients die in the field, some in the emergency department, some make it to the operating room and die on the table, and some make it to us.

But the fight for their life isn't over when they get to the SICU. A few may die here, and some may recover, but most will never be the same, neither physically nor psychologically. Some will be left paralyzed, unable to ever care for themselves again. There will be some, even some as young as 16, who will be left forever bedbound. These people are given a breathing and feeding tube, and are transferred to a long-term care facility; they are likely to return with complications. Some are brain damaged as a result of their injuries and are also transferred to a long-term care facility, where they will probably remain bed-bound for the rest of their lives.

The more fortunate ones recover and go to a rehabilitation facility, or even go home. I tell them that we have managed their wounds this time, but next time we may not be able to do so. I tell them, "The tough part is on you now, make sure you don't risk your life and put yourself in danger again." I advise them to move and get out of these crime-infested neighborhoods. But it is not so simple when their circumstances hold them hostage to these neighborhoods and their street laws. This is what they were born into, this is where they grew up, and this is the only way they know.

Near my ZIP code, the hospitals are expanding. They are being bought up and becoming part of a chain of a massive healthcare system. But here, in the roughest and most dangerous neighborhoods of Chicago, where the need is greatest, hospitals are shutting down.

The Challenges of Practicing Scientific Medicine

Scientific medicine has been a detrimental development in regards to the poorer classes in society. Racial minorities in particular have been excluded from entering the profession, while their traditional medicine is no longer accessible to them.[16]

As the emphasis on medical education has grown, so has the cost of pursuing it. As the bar to graduate with an MD degree kept rising, many previous candidates were eliminated, and fewer doctors were being produced. As the number of doctors decreased, the demand grew exponentially, further widening the gap in health education and its increasingly complicated healthcare system.

With the decreased number of doctors, a new need arose to divide and delegate their previous roles and responsibilities down the chain of medical professionals, such as nursing. New advanced degrees were created to divide the roles and supply the demand, without increasing the number of doctors, whose high pay is secured by their low numbers. Their income security is deemed necessary to cover the high costs of their increasingly high student loan debt, and the loss of potential income during their extensive years of study.

The Complexity of Role Division

It is no longer a single physician who has gotten to know their patients on an intimate level, with their relationship developed over many years of practice at a community clinic. That doctor has since been replaced by a team of professionals like Physician Assistants (PA), Nurse Practitioners (NP), Registered Nurses (RN), Licensed Practical Nurses (LPN), Patient Care Technicians (PCT), Certified Nurses Assistants (CNA) and Medical Assistants (MA).

---

16 Brown, 2017.

For children born in low socioeconomic ZIP codes, to become a doctor is close to impossible. Even for the brightest minds, who manage to get recognized and are given scholarships, the reality of these neighborhoods and the laws of division based on property tax are difficult to escape. Even at elementary level, the standardized tests that assess reading, math, and science skills show many high-income students fall within the 75th to 90th percentiles or higher. Low-income students, on the other hand, score in the bottom quartile, indicating that they perform at a level 25% below that of their peers nationally. [17]

Illiteracy

This concerning statistic became a reality for me when one of my patients underwent a tracheostomy procedure after he'd been shot. We needed to create an alternative airway in his neck, allowing him to get off the ventilator. The patient was in his 40s and had grown up in the local community. He was not able to use his voice to communicate his needs and, after a few attempts to read his lips without much progress, and increased frustration for us both, I handed him a clipboard with paper and a pencil to write them down instead. That's when I realized he couldn't read or write. He was very kind and cooperative, but his inability to write proved to be a huge hindrance in his new situation. Using a writing pad for patients who have undergone tracheostomy, our standard practice, was not available to him.

Since then, our admission assessment questions pertaining to literacy, one I've often skipped by assuming the answer was obvious – "Do you know how to read and write?" – has gained an entirely new meaning and value. It's one I don't allow myself to skip anymore.

The Street Laws

Children in these low-income communities, stigmatized by their ZIP code, don't have the same family support as children who grow up in better

---

[17] National Center for Education & Statistics; NCES.ed.gov.

neighborhoods. They are often sent to school to get the free high-calorie low-nutrient lunch, rather than to get an education. These children are often discouraged from aspiring to a higher level of education since not only does it cost the parents a lot of money, but also prevents them from earning money and relieving the family, struggling to make ends meet, from its financial burden.

Social status and success in these neighborhoods is gained by the ability to earn money as early and as quickly as possible. How doesn't matter, as long as it's enough for the family. The level of income to qualify for public aid such as food stamps, supplemental housing, and free insurance is impossible to live off. To avoid losing these benefits, members will supplement the family income through illegal work.

I remember asking another patient, recovering from a traumatic injury caused by multiple gunshot wounds, what he could do to prevent a similar future trauma. He worked as a security guard, who supplemented his low income by selling illicit drugs. He was puzzled. After all, he was selling on his corner and in his territory. He couldn't believe the disrespect he had gotten. "Seems like both the street laws and the drugs are nothing like they used to be," I responded.

Struggling for food, and dealing with unstable family dynamics, not to mention abuse and neglect – how can the children of these communities become empowered to move up the ZIP code? As our educational and technological advancements in medicine grow, so do the socioeconomic gaps in our society. Fewer people in low-income ZIP codes have access to care, except in cases of life-threatening emergencies, like trauma as a result of gun violence. In fact, many have never even had a home-cooked meal.

Teaching vs Primary Care Hospitals

As an ICU nurse, I have experience of two very different structures within the hospital system one, a safety net teaching hospital; the other, a primary care physician facility.

Teaching hospitals are often located in the inner cities and are affiliated with universities. They provide opportunities for medical students and residents to practice and learn. On the other hand, primary care hospitals are often located on the outskirts of cities, or in rural areas. They are community hospitals where attending doctors have the sole responsibility for managing patient care. Each system has its benefits and problems; but in both systems we see how doctors are becoming managers in the care of their patients, rather than providing care directly to them.

That means in practice, based on my own experience, what was once the physician's role of providing direct care to patients is now carried out by nurses or other healthcare practitioners. These days, doctors spend most of their time at computers, reading through their patients' charts, which include diagnostic imaging and laboratory test results, as well as reviewing information from all previous visits and hospitalizations. Considering how sick our general population has become, and how specialized our care has gotten, they have a vast amount of material to process. As a result, mistakes can be made. Adverse events, harmful outcomes occurring during medical care, are now affecting at least one in ten patients.[18]

Increased Productivity?

The number of physicians has decreased and the complexity of caring for our sick patients has increased. Direct patient care has been delegated to nurses and other bedside professionals.

Have you ever been a patient in the hospital, or perhaps had a family member who has been a patient, and asked to see the doctor? It's getting harder to see one. The reason is that there isn't just one doctor taking care of you; there are many, depending on your condition. Furthermore, they do not reside in the hospitals as they have their clinics to run. They see their patients once a day on their "rounds," and if you want to see your doctor you'd better not miss that once-a-day chance. Don't even think to ask what time that will be, since the doctors themselves often don't know.

---

[18] Skelly et al., 2022.

As much as the patients want to see their doctors, this is a problem for their nurses too. Speaking as the one providing direct care, I can't tell you how often I've been frustrated by this situation. I have often gathered questions from my patients and their families – as well as having had my own – and waited for a particular physician, only to find out that they have already been on their rounds. They had reviewed the chart, put in their note, and left without a word.

I understand that they are often so overwhelmed with their workload that they might not be able to see me, but I am a valuable resource in patient care. Intensive Care Unit (ICU) nurses check on their patients every hour, answer the families' calls, and respond to the patients' call lights. They do physical assessments and reassess every two hours. Nurses administer medications, carry out the physicians' orders, and take patients for their diagnostic testing. They clean, bathe, feed, and dress wounds. Nurses develop an intimate relationship with their patients and their families, a relationship which is difficult to reflect in a computer note.

This complex practice of scientific medicine has changed the role of doctors and of other medical professions. Nursing is becoming increasingly threatened with the same problem; we spend less and less time with our patients. ICU documentation is so lengthy that we can be sitting at a computer throughout our entire shift, in order to meet the mandatory requirements of the hospital. Patients have a hard time getting to see their doctors, but more often, they are upset because of waiting too long to see their nurse.

As a result of this emerging problem and to spread awareness, an initiative called "Leave Nurses at the Bedside" was established. Installing computers in every room of the ICU was one of the innovations of that initiative.

One of the benefits of this approach is that it allows for real-time documentation. We can scan medications at our patients' bedsides, significantly improving medication safety. On the downside, nurses now have a computer between themselves and the patient. I have found myself taking notes while I am interacting with the patient, in an attempt to save time. This depersonalized way of interaction further impedes the nurse-patient relationship and disrupts the intimate one-on-one space where true healing is likely to take place.

Working in the ICU is stressful due to the severity of our patients' conditions, but another factor in this stress is time management. You can't provide the best care if it isn't timely, and if you haven't finished your documentation, you can't go home at the end of your 12-hour shift. You must stay on to record all of your interventions. If the patient was so sick that providing care meant you didn't have time to document at all, you have that much more to catch up on. On one of my worst shifts, I remember staying on for four extra hours, extending the hours I worked that day to 16. I still had to work my scheduled 12-hour shift the next day.

The Art and Science of Nursing

I loved studying the human body when I was in college. I still remember my first physiology class, in which, by the use of big, colorful puzzles, the teacher taught us the intricate details of peptides and how they all fit together to make a protein. My jaw dropped and only closed again once class was over. I was hypnotized by the logic of human creation. What a wonder we all are! The body's intelligence is remarkable.

At college, Mr. William Andresen was the best anatomy and physiology teacher one could wish for. His highly-ranked recognition among the students made his classes so popular that they would fill up immediately. The workload was intense so about 40% would later drop out, mostly within the first two weeks. But the determined ones recognized the value of an incredible teacher. To register for his classes, students would line up hours before the start of registration, even before the school had opened. Computer in hand, we would start to line up as early as 3:00 to be certain that we could get in. This was the most secure way. If the school server froze, you would still be able to register in person. That is, only if you took the time to secure your spot in line early enough.

He was a humble, approachable man who truly appreciated how the human body works, and he shared that passion with his students in the most expressive of ways. He wouldn't just read from his premade slides; instead, he would draw pictures and diagrams to help us connect the intricate details of human physiology. Or he would get on top of a stool and dangle his arms and legs like a mannequin to explain joints, tendons, and ligaments. From his office window, impossible to miss, overlooked a gigantic plush green and yellow frog. It was his way of paying tribute to the species we used for learning anatomy and physiology. I loved going to his classes.

I was equally fortunate with my microbiology and sociology teachers. They made the class content so enjoyable that studying it was nearly effortless. You couldn't help but pay attention.

Unfortunately, my experience in nursing school was a different story. That passion for learning, which I had while studying science, and my excitement at becoming a nurse, was brutally destroyed by the teacher nurses and the confusion evoked by their subjective exam questions. If the majority of the class initially failed an exam, their scores would be revised to increase the class average, in order for most to pass and continue in the nursing program.

Throughout the entire nursing program, we were kept on the verge of failing Studying and preparing for nursing exams was nothing like it had been when I studied anatomy and physiology. Many exam questions had different possible answers. To pass, it was necessary to develop a skill in answering convoluted questions. This created unnecessary stress and competition among the nursing students, who became reluctant even to share their study materials.

Which Answer is Right?

When friends in nursing school put some of their test questions to me, I still can't get the "right" answer, despite my 14 years of clinical practice as a nurse. Take this question for example:

SCIENTIFIC MEDICINE

You are caring for a client who has had a right-sided stroke and is currently on aspiration precaution and receiving all medication via Duotube. Your client develops an elevated temperature (102 F) that requires you to administer ibuprofen. Please answer both parts of this question to receive full credit.

Order: 600mg ibuprofen every 8 hours for temperature greater than 101.5 F

On hand: 200mg ibuprofen tablets or ibuprofen liquid, 500mg/1 tsp.

First, answer which ibuprofen option you would administer via Duotube—tablets or liquid?

Second, depending on your first answer, identify how many tablets per dose or what ml. dose you would administer.

Duotube is a feeding tube that allows for the administering of medications or liquid food to patients with compromised swallowing ability; as in this case, after a stroke. Medications in pill form are crushed and mixed in water to make them liquid, so that they can be administered through a tube, such as Duotube. Some medications should not be crushed, but ibuprofen is not one of them. Pills are less expensive, and so, in this scenario, administering 3 x 200mg pills is time-efficient and has a much lower margin for error. It is easy and practical. No need to complicate things, right?

Wrong! The approved answer is liquid.

Let's put this test answer in a real-life scenario. The question does not state what unit this patient is in, or how many more patients you are taking care of at the time, or how critical their conditions are. The question makes no mention of these circumstances but, in the real world, they are extremely relevant.

Imagine that this patient is still in the ICU and their fever spiked at the same time as your other patient is not doing well. The other patient is on a ventilator and their oxygen saturation is going down, so their ventilation requirements are being adjusted.

All of a sudden you have multiple orders to carry out and coordinate. One of them is an emergency CT scan, so as to rule out a pulmonary embolism. You have called the CT team to let them know you're on the way. The respiratory team and the transport team are all ready to go, but you want to administer this ibuprofen before you leave, so it starts working while you are gone. In these real-life circumstances, would you stop to calculate the right amount of liquid, or grab 3 tablets of Ibuprofen?

Even if you chose the liquid dose, would you be able to find a syringe with a tsp measurement on it? If not, it is impossible to accurately administer 1.2 tsp. As a practitioner, I would always choose to give the pills in the above scenario. Therefore, I would most likely fail this exam, even after many years of nursing practice. There isn't just one correct answer to these questions.

The explanation for the approved answer is that the pill form, if not crushed and mixed thoroughly, may clog up the tube, so the liquid form is less risky. Perhaps that explanation would make more sense to me if all feeding tube medications were supplied in a liquid form, but most of them are pills that need to be crushed and dissolved before administration. From my years of practice, I would say that performing calculations, finding an appropriate syringe with desired markings, and drawing the exact amount is far more time-consuming and has far greater potential for error.

Nurse Kasia's tip: when mixing and administering medications through a tube, first pour warm water into a little medication cup containing the crushed meds, then allow it to dissolve while performing your many other tasks. This makes drawing up the softened, and already partly dissolved, medications into a piston syringe so much easier. Next, pull back on the plunger to get some air into the syringe, put your finger over the hub, and give it a good mix. Swirling the syringe while administering the medication through a tube is another way to ensure that sediment does not accumulate at the bottom, and therefore doesn't clog up the tube.

Importance of Real-Life Experience

Practice makes all the difference, yet the emphasis in nursing schools is placed elsewhere. The above example of a nursing exam question is confusing. Instead of confusing our nursing students with subjective exam questions, why can't we make sure they feel competent in their nursing skills at the time of their graduation? Importantly, knowledge of anatomy, physiology, pathophysiology, and microbiology must be allied with practical nursing skills. Nursing students must be allowed to practice these skills safely, enabling them to transfer their textbook knowledge to the bedside. Time management, as well as critical and functional thinking, is of utmost importance and can't be mastered through the mind alone. It would be like trying to master different forms of martial arts by reading books and watching videos. Simply impossible. In nursing, just as in martial arts, most of us can memorize rules and the reasoning behind them, but only through years of practice can we actually master them.

For this reason, nursing is considered both an art and a science.

Currently, nurses, especially nurse practitioners, are given the responsibilities of filling gaps caused by the shortage of physicians. They are expected to make critical decisions that require extensive medical knowledge and training. But, as demonstrated by the nursing exam question above, they are not receiving the necessary preparation, nor do the test questions adequately reflect the gravity and complexity of the responsibilities they are faced with.

Nursing students need more clinical hours and greater exposure to real-life situations. However, the current process of providing clinical training requires significant improvement. Nursing schools typically establish affiliation agreements with hospitals, but the bedside nurses responsible for training students are not included in these agreements. On clinical days, nursing instructors bring groups of five to seven students into the hospital and attempt to pair them with bedside nurses across different units. This placement process has become increasingly difficult, as many nurses—

already overwhelmed by heavy workloads and the responsibility of training new hires—are reluctant to take on students who require extra attention and may slow them down.

As a result, clinical instructors often struggle to secure meaningful placements, leaving students without the hands-on experience they need. Nurses, when asked to take a student at the last minute, feel pressured and frustrated. At the same time, declining a student can leave them feeling guilty. This unnecessary frustration could be avoided with a structured system in place. Bedside nurses should be incentivized and properly compensated for training students. Additionally, they need advance notice and dedicated time to commit to teaching, rather than being approached on the day of training in front of the instructor and student—an awkward situation that can leave students feeling rejected.

Reflecting on my nursing education, the focus was on instilling medical knowledge while emphasizing that we were not physicians. However, in practice, nurses are clinical practitioners who are often expected to make critical decisions requiring a level of medical knowledge and expertise comparable to that of physicians. We were taught that nurses do not diagnose medical conditions. A nurse wouldn't state that a patient has pneumonia – that's a medical diagnosis. Instead, her nursing diagnosis would be somewhere along the lines of "impaired gas exchange related to alveolar-capillary membrane changes, inflammation, or fluid in the lungs as evidenced by hypoxia (low oxygen saturation), dyspnea (difficulty breathing), cyanosis (bluish skin) or restlessness." You tell me which one sounds easier.

Effective nurses must be able to detect symptoms of disease and signs of deterioration at an early stage, so that appropriate interventions can quickly take place. They must also know what these appropriate interventions are, so that they can effectively advocate or intervene. Nurses need a high level of medical knowledge, and to have had opportunities to implement their nursing skills, so as to effectively care for their patients.

SCIENTIFIC MEDICINE

Computerize the Job, Depersonalize the Care

Computers are beneficial tools when it comes to communication and management, but healthcare providers are spending too much time on them. Computers help us to organize our tasks and are excellent for gathering and evaluating data.

I appreciate computers and the internet for the way they have expanded our knowledge and transformed our lives. However, all this technology does not come without a price. Nursing has become so task-oriented that we forget the bigger picture and no longer do we see the patient as a person. With the aid of computers, healthcare has become planned out to the last detail. No time is allowed for interacting with patients or responding when they press their call-light buttons. Nurses now are often too busy, so hospitals hire certified nursing assistants (CNA) or patient care technicians (PCT) – the name says it all! – to assist with patients' needs and answering call lights. Delegating patients' care down the line to other providers is another manifestation of the increasing demands and complexity of modern healthcare. Physicians delegate to nurses, nurses to nursing assistants. Soon it may be as rare to see a nurse come to the bedside as is now the case with physicians.

Caregiver Shortage, Administration Surplus

With the long-predicted nursing shortage has come the increase of administrative positions and the growing "chain of command". I have been experiencing this phenomenon throughout my nursing practice. No longer does the unit have a charge nurse, manager, and director; now we boast a PCC (patient care coordinator), a CCC (clinical care coordinator), an HA (house administrator), and HOC (house operation coordinator). It has gotten so complicated that it is difficult to remember all the differences between these job descriptions and their responsibilities. This is to say nothing of the new administrative positions and titles constantly being created and redefined.

More concerning is the shortage of nurses to provide proper 24-hour bedside care, not to mention those nurses who now take on administrative roles. Because bedside nursing is very demanding, resulting in burnout, these executive positions can be seen as an alternative career path. But if nursing skills are not kept up, as with all other skills, they become difficult, or even impossible, to perform. This means that in times of critical urgency, these administrator nurses would not be able (or perhaps some would not choose) to step into the role of a bedside care provider. Tension, conflict, resistance, and division between bedside nurses and the administration abound as a result.

Everything is interconnected, and everything produces consequences. The computers on which we have come to depend gather masses of data that has to be reviewed and analyzed, taking up a lot of time and effort. Doctors or nursing supervisors evaluate the data and develop interventions. Based on the information gathered, doctors place orders for each particular patient. At the same time, nursing supervisors, or hospital administrative workers, gather different data: about a hospital unit, say, or the overall performance of an entire hospital. This data reflects such things as patient satisfaction scores and infection rates.

Unrealistic Goals

Bedside nurses must respond both to doctor orders and to management directives. Because of the growing disconnect from the bedside, some of these orders, interventions, or goals are unrealistic.

For example, some diagnostic tests ordered on critical patients may carry risks that outweigh their benefits. The diagnostic test may provide extra information and seem, after reviewing the patient's chart, to be a good idea. In reality, this documentation may not reveal the full extent of the patient's instability, observed at the bedside throughout the shift. The trip itself may carry risks that further compromise the patient's safety. Nurses are responsible for speaking up and advocating in these situations.

These unrealistic expectations and unrealistic interventions are a sign of detachment from the bedside and its reality – on the part of doctors, nursing supervisors, and hospital administrators. It is all very well for a doctor to order an upper gastro-intestinal study when they have never actually poured a liter or more of contrast through the nasogastric tube of a sick patient with an already distended abdomen. Those physicians who are doing the ordering are not there to witness the excruciating pain suffered by the patient after each dose. They don't see, or clean up the vomit, that often results from this procedure.

An example of an unrealistic intervention directed by management requires nurses to answer call lights within two minutes – to raise patient satisfaction scores. I remember 12-hour shifts during which I was too busy to take a lunch break. I would be out of the unit for much of that shift, taking one of my patients to have a diagnostic test. On returning to the unit, I would still have to catch up on my other patient. At the end of one particular shift, while catching up on all the documentation, I was approached by the nurse in charge. A paper was handed to me to sign as proof that I was notified that my patient's call light was not answered within the two-minute time frame. I tried to explain that I wasn't even on the unit, but I was told that I was ultimately responsible, since it was my patient's call light.

Often, there aren't enough nurses to safely cover for those having lunch, or taking a patient for diagnostic testing. Taking on another nurse's patient or patients, on top of one's own, is not safe, and should never be considered as such. I understand that patient satisfaction scores are important, and answering call lights in a timely manner is necessary; but also important is the well-being of nurses and their job satisfaction, because they are the ones making it all happen.

Balancing the numbers by leaving a unit short-staffed results in pain and suffering for those who can't advocate for themselves. It is easy for management to forget that the numbers on their grid are human patients. The nurses will survive these shifts, but their patients may not.

Chapter 3

The Sick-Care Model

Our Disease-Focused System

> *Out of this social intervention perspective and the charity organization movement emerged the social work professions. Case workers, settlement house workers, correctional administrators, probation officers, and their academic advisers shared with the middle and upper classes the prevailing social Darwinist view that dependent poverty, crime, and social deviance in general had biological roots. But this new professional class believed that medical and social intervention could remedy 'natural' imperfections.[19]*
>
> Dr. E. Richard Brown

As we have already seen, the idea that disease is the cause of all evil suited the most influential class in society. But fundamental aspects concerning health and healing were overlooked. Blinded by arrogance, our leaders refused to see the true complexity of the matter. Healing, defined by Professor Quinn in *The Art and Science of Nurse Coaching*, as "an emergent process of the whole system, bringing together aspects of oneself and the body-mind-spirit-environment-culture-society at a more profound level of inner knowing,"[20] was conveniently dismissed.

In other words, healing comes from not only our environment and our culture but also the body, mind, and spirit of each individual within it.[21] But this more profound approach was disregarded. It was much easier to say that all our health problems are down to disease and to use science and technology to fix them. As a result, we began applying layer upon layer of scientific and technological camouflage to hide the social issues that such a disease-focused system may never resolve.

---

19 Brown, 2017.
20 Southard et al., 2020.
21 Southard et al., 2020.

If, instead of focusing on biological causes and natural imperfections, we had looked deeper into the structures of the society we have built, relating this to cultures and behavior, we could have gotten nearer to the root of the problem.

We would have then been able to look at crime, not only as an imperfection but also as an adaptation to poverty. Social deviance could be seen as an adaptation to trauma, and sickness and disease as manifestations of conflict. Our inability to resolve social issues lies not in our lack of intelligence, but in our lack of compassion. This is how our society misunderstands, or perhaps chooses to misunderstand, the problems we create.

The Holistic View

Perhaps we got it all wrong and, instead of looking for ways to fix our biological nature, we should search for ways not to destroy it; instead of treating it as a blunder, we should cherish it as the miracle that it is. This approach could transform our healthcare system from "sick" care to "health" care. To do that health must be treated holistically, not merely focusing on human anatomy, but considering all aspects of our living experience. We must see past ourselves, honoring all life, all living things, since our health or well-being can never be isolated or separate from the life of another.

To put this in a global context: Cutting down forests disrupts the health of our planet, which results in climate changes, leading to more frequent natural disasters. Laws of ownership and exploitation of land and its natural resources create great inequalities, and these affect us all. Laws designed to protect nature and the well-being of our planet should be strengthened. Our forests would not then be cut down simply for the financial profit of an individual or company. As for society: Instead of punishing crime and expanding penitentiaries, we should focus more on prevention. Providing guidance and support to stay-at-home mothers caring for our future generations would build strong communities. The result: a safe and well-cared-for society will exhibit less disease.

Blinded by self-interest, we fail to see the unity of all creation. What should be first and foremost? We fail to see the unity of mind, body, and spirit within ourselves. We fail to see connections: neighbors with foreigners, forests with houses. We fail to see the interdependence of the entire cosmos.

The truth is, we fail to see the bigger picture. We are unable to recognize that if we do wrong to others, it will rebound on ourselves. We wouldn't need to be so consumed with **fixing** our world if we stopped **destroying** it in the first place.

If we looked harder, we would see an intricate relationship between our actions and the root causes of many diseases. Nature is not the culprit. Yes, we may be genetically predisposed to certain characteristics, but by treating our human nature, our genes, and our physical bodies, without acknowledging the immense impact of our thoughts, perceptions, and beliefs, we fail to realize that this path can only lead to a dead end.

Quick Fixes

Poverty can be alleviated by social workers, substitute housing, and food stamps, but it can't be fixed by them alone. Crime will not be resolved solely by correctional administrators, probationary officers, and penitentiaries. In the same way, our unsustainable healthcare system can't be fixed just by technology. Type II diabetes is not eliminated by insulin, nor is autoimmunity cured by steroids.

These quick fixes, as wonderful as they are in times of crisis, are not resolutions to the complex issues at hand. They may control the situation, but they also reinforce the inequality of the situation. Who is applying the quick fixes? Who is applying the band-aid over these deep wounds? It may make a government or an individual/entity feel better because they are doing something, but one side is patching up while the other is in need and dependent.

To fix poverty, crime, and disease, we must see how we continue to create it. You may be wondering why I say "we" and feel like I'm being unfair, but the truth is that our society is only a reflection of what goes on between each and every one of us. We are all part of the solution, and we all have the ability to respond. The more aware we ourselves become, the more thoughtful our choices can be. If enough of us realize and make small changes, a major shift will start happening.

Accept, Unite, Include

The way we nourish our bodies, perceive different situations, feel about ourselves and others – all this expresses health or it expresses disease. Our life experiences can influence our genetic makeup through a process called epigenetics. Everything is interconnected and interrelated. If you change your own experience through awareness, you could change your gene expression, and that of your future generations! This is called epigenetic inheritance.

If, for example, you are in a stressful situation but do not feel stressed, you could be avoiding harmful long-term effects such as inflammation, and any associated negative gene expression. Or imagine you are on your dream vacation, or getting married to the one you love. Instead of enjoying the moment, you worry over minor details you have no control over. This also may evoke physiological damage by way of the stress you are feeling. Perception is key.

The remnants of that same sick-care model that originated long ago with Rockefeller and Gates, evolving over the years, is what we practice in medicine today. Previously, I analyzed the fragmentation of hospital roles into bedside care and management. I also talked about the social injustice which exists in our practice of medicine, between doctor and patient; and I have pointed to the detachment of ourselves both from our human nature and from each other.

Let us no longer detach, but accept. Unite, rather than divide. Include, not exclude.

Instead of fighting our nature, let's embrace it and, by discovering which of our actions leads to disease, prevent it.

Dividing the Body

It is astonishing how our bodies have evolved to become so complex. It may appear simple since much of the body's intense work seems entirely effortless; but if we try to understand how it works, it is extremely difficult. In investigating all of the physiological, biochemical, microbiological, and other reactions that are needed for the simplest of our body's tasks, we reach the limits of our intellect. Discoveries are being made daily, which allow us to understand how different parts of the body relate to and depend on each other. The more we discover, the more we realize that everything is connected. Within the body, nothing goes unnoticed.

Constantly, in each of us, all of these involuntary and complex reactions are performed independently of our consciousness. It can take the mind a lifetime to comprehend what the body does in an instant.

Within medicine there now exist specialties and subspecialties. It is too much for one person to research and be an expert on the entire body, so we now have experts in cardiology, neurology, gynecology, nephrology (kidneys), to name but a few.

All the parts and systems of the body, all of its different organs, and all of the diseases from which it may suffer – each has a corresponding specialty. But, in understanding the body and making sense of it, our knowledge has become fragmented. Despite our best efforts, we have divided our understanding, and we may fail to recognize that best practice is not possible through division. That we should have to divide up our knowledge of the body in this way should make us humble. Instead, as experts in one small area, we become self-righteous and ignorant.

Furthermore, in the words of that tireless advocate for health reform, Dr. Richard Brown, "*specialization among practitioners was encouraged by economic competition within the profession.*"[22]

Specialization in Practice

In my own nursing practice, I have experienced two different types of Intensive Care Unit (ICU) – the closed unit and the open. In a "closed" unit, which I encountered at a teaching hospital, a final decision is made by the resident doctor and his supervising attending physician, having consulted different specialists and receiving their recommendations. The "open" ICU was at a primary care hospital that doesn't have residents since it's not a teaching facility. In this case, on being consulted, each doctor gives their own orders for each of their ICU patients. One patient can have five or more attending doctors writing orders. An ICU "intensivist" stays on the unit but does not necessarily see all of the patients on the unit. It depends on whether they were consulted, and if this sounds confusing, that's because it is.

I have never been able to understand why the ICU intensivist doctor, the only doctor to stay on the unit, isn't consulted on each and every patient within the unit. I would go into their office asking for urgent or straightforward orders, only to hear their "I'm not on the case" response, which was frustrating and infuriating. It seems so simple: the patient needs immediate help! But unfortunately, that's not how the system works. It's another form of detachment. Bureaucracy takes precedence over patient needs.

Protocols

Legally, bedside nurses cannot prescribe medicines or order treatment, but they MUST react immediately and appropriately. How they do this is defined by protocols (procedures), specific to particular situations that

---

22   Brown, 2017.

might be experienced by their patients. ICUs are full of rules for nurses to follow. There are strict guidelines that they must observe. Nurses are legally responsible for knowing these protocols and implementing them.

Protocols enable nurses to run ICUs without doctors present. Most procedures ordered by the doctors are already included in these protocols, but sometimes they are not. Things get complicated and stressful for the nurse when a patient needs a time-sensitive intervention that nurses can immediately identify, but for which no order has been written. Immediate attention doesn't allow time to page the doctors and wait for their response. In these circumstances, nurses may administer emergency medications without a pre-existing order, but that order must then be placed within 15 minutes.

There are also "standing orders" or "order sets" that are given on admission of a patient to the ICU. The nurses must page the physician for any other orders that are not part of any protocol. In a non-teaching setting, after getting the physician's approval, the nurses are often asked to put the orders in the computer themselves, under that physician's name. These are called "verbal orders," to be used in emergencies only, but in reality, commonly practiced.

As an ICU nurse, I must recognize that my patient needs immediate attention, know what to do about it, notify the physician, put the required orders in for that physician, and carry them out promptly. Sound stressful? Let's not forget about my other patient. Their call light might be going off, and remember, it must be answered within two minutes; at the same time addressing the life-threatening issues of my first patient, crashing in another room.

Increasing Pressure on Nurses

This current dysfunctional healthcare system is now pressuring nurses to do things beyond their scope of practice, like putting physician orders in. By law, that practice should only be applied in emergencies but, especially in non-teaching hospitals, it has become the norm. Physicians are too busy to put their orders in, which is then defaulted on to the nurses to do it for them. If the physicians are "too busy," so are the nurses, or more so.

When nurses advocate for more autonomy, they don't want more power or responsibility – they want to legalize what they are already doing so that they don't lose their nursing license.

Another problem nurses are facing in this divided system is that of conflicting orders issued by different doctors. For example, a cardiologist may order medications that lower the patient's blood pressure, but at the same time compromise the health of that patient's kidneys, resulting in kidney failure and putting that patient on dialysis. Medication doses require constant revisions since ICU patients' conditions are volatile. The cardiologist is not always there to witness these emerging changes, so nurses need to be vigilant.

At times, as I have said, the cardiologist and the nephrologist may write orders that are at odds with one another. One specialist may write orders to stop IV fluids to take strain off the heart, while the other specialist orders more IV fluids, to increase the perfusion to the kidneys and prevent them from failing. Each doctor is fighting to protect their particular organ. Which one to choose, the heart or the kidneys? Or perhaps, the lungs or the heart? The brain or the kidneys? Which one would you choose?

Removal of organs: Organectomy

What about all the other organs that lack reputation? They serve no real purpose, anyway. Take them out! What's the big deal? Recurrent infections of the tonsils? Tonsillectomy. Inflamed appendix or appendicitis? Appendectomy. Inflamed gallbladder or cholecystitis? cholecystectomy. Heavy or painful menstruation after childbirth? hysterectomy. Preventing pregnancy after childbirth? salpingectomy. Back problems? laminectomy. So on and so forth. Even the patients themselves ask the doctors: Do I need it? Can you take it out?

The body is a miracle that we continue to study and, despite our technological advances, still cannot fully comprehend. Yet we treat it with such ignorance.

With each organ we take out, we take no account of the subtle messages the body uses to communicate imbalance. Knowledge of healing in unity with the body's energies, such as *Nadi* in Indian medicine, and *Chi* in Chinese medicine, is unacknowledged in the West.

Natural Medicine

Ayurveda, a natural system of medicine from India, derives its name from the Sanskrit words *ayur* (life) and *veda* (science or knowledge). Nadi, in Ayurvedic medicine, refers to energy channels or pathways through which a life force, called *prana*, flows through the body.[23] The balance and unimpeded flow of prana through the nadis is essential for overall health and well-being. Ayurvedic practices, such as yoga and meditation, aim to balance and harmonize the flow of energy in the nadis.

Similarly, *Chi* or *Qi* in Traditional Chinese Medicine (TCM) is the vital energy or life force that flows through the meridians or channels in the body. There are 12 main meridians, and numerous smaller ones, each associated with specific organs and functions. Acupuncture, acupressure, herbal medicine, tai chi and qigong are some of the practices in TCM aimed at maintaining the balance and proper flow of chi.

Both Ayurveda and TCM emphasize the importance of balance and free-flowing energy for maintaining health and preventing illness. Lovers of Star Wars will remember the phrase, "May the Force be with you." The idea of life force energy and its essence is something we relate to, since so much of what we experience in life cannot be explained by the logical mind.

Yet despite this intuitive longing for balance in our lives, the radical interventions of conventional medicine, with its invasive procedures, and

---

23   There are 72,000 nadis, of which three main ones called Ida, Pingala, and Sushumna, are considered most significant.

the consequent formation of scar tissue, impede this balance. While natural remedies like herbal supplements and homeopathic medications have been the basis of many pharmaceuticals, their value has been denied. Instead, their synthetic versions, and the technical skill of surgical interventions, are given credit.

There is a long history of medical doctors opposing homeopathy. Homeopathy directly competed with mainstream medicine. This competition led physicians' organizations to take action against homeopathic practitioners. In 1860, the Massachusetts Medical Society started barring homeopaths from membership. During the 1870s, the American Medical Association (AMA) spearheaded a broader offensive against homeopathy and other alternative medical practices viewed as "operating outside of mainstream medicine."

The AMA's ethical code prohibited physicians from consulting with practitioners of these "sectarian" or unorthodox medical systems, as well as with female or Black doctors, who faced discrimination and exclusion from the medical establishment at that time.[24]

Are Unimportant Organs Important?

Surgical interventions and technological advancements save many lives. Indeed, these skills are irreplaceable, and crucial in case of a traumatic injury or congenital defects. But, in many other cases, invasive procedures can be avoided with dietary or lifestyle changes, and by the practice of preventative or holistic (functional) medicine.

Removing an organ without diagnosing the root cause of the disorder may result in life-long side effects. Scars arising from surgery may obstruct the energy flow of our nadis or our chi. If they are particularly large, or located near important energy channels, we should try to avoid them. The organ that surgery would remove is one part of an entire system in which everything is interconnected. Healing an organ, rather than removing

---

24 Brown, 2017.

it, may make a difference in the whole system. Perhaps that organ is communicating an imbalance affecting the body, which should prompt us to change. Removing this troublesome organ may make the problem go away, but will only dissuade us from making necessary lifestyle changes, and we may become sicker in the long run.

Only recently have these "unimportant organs" started to gain some attention and appreciation. For example, new scientific discoveries are being made on the importance of our microbiome, which are the microscopic organisms that live inside us. It turns out that their presence is a much greater marker of our overall health than we had realized. We need them, balanced and in large numbers, to stay healthy. Corporations now make millions of dollars talking up "pro" and "pre" biotics, and it turns out that one of their homes is the appendix, amongst other places. Even though you may live without your appendix, you will have fewer of these essential creatures protecting you.

Gallbladder pain may signify a more complex issue with the liver; therefore, removal should not be taken lightly. Biliary sludge is a mixture of bile, cholesterol crystals, and calcium salts that can form in the gallbladder and bile ducts, causing gallbladder inflammation or cholecystitis. Some examples of the conditions of the liver that may alter bile composition are Primary Sclerosing Cholangitis (PSC), Liver Cirrhosis, and Non-Alcoholic Fatty Liver Disease (NAFLD), associated with metabolic syndrome, obesity, and diabetes.

Gallstones from diabetes-related changes like poor glucose control can lead to cholecystitis. Removal of the gallbladder addresses the immediate problem, but it does not address the underlying obesity or diabetes, which can cause recurrent issues. High cholesterol levels may also lead to the formation of gallstones. While surgery to remove the gallbladder addresses the immediate gallstone problem, the underlying hyperlipidemia (high cholesterol and triglycerides) often remains unaddressed. This can continue to affect liver health and pose a significant risk for heart and vascular diseases.

Hysterectomy may trigger premature menopause, associated with several health risks and premature aging. Even the disposal of our wisdom teeth to keep the rest nice and straight may have much greater significance than we previously realized. Smaller jaws may affect our breathing and be linked to sleep apnea.

Science is constantly changing and continually being revised in the light of new evidence. We should be humbled by these discoveries rather than ignoring them.

Increasing knowledge should keep us open-minded and grateful for all the new treatment opportunities that arise. But old wisdom and ancient remedies don't always have to be replaced with recent technological advancements. Why limit ourselves? There is no one way to stay healthy. We would do better to refrain from judgment, as closing ourselves off to alternatives may ultimately work to our own disadvantage.

Treating the Symptoms Rather Than Finding the Cause

Our current lifestyle has turned healthcare into sick-care. We neglect our health, become ill as a result, and then treat the symptoms, rather than finding the root cause and addressing the fundamental problem of why we got sick in the first place. Why not look at the imbalance that we have created ourselves? A better course of treatment would be to look at the entire body and its environment holistically; they are connected with each other. Instead, our approach is fragmented; our medicine is divided.

In our society, where "productivity above all" is the motto, we are forgetting how to take care of our health:

Tired? *Drink coffee.*

Exhausted? *Drink coffee and take Adderall.*

Acid reflux? *Drink coffee but take a Tums with it. If that doesn't help, ask your doctor for Nexium or Prilosec.*

High blood sugar and diabetes? *Take Metformin and insulin.*

Blood pressure issues? *No problem. So many choices! How about Lisinopril, Metoprolol, or Amlodipine?*

High cholesterol? *We've got statins! There's nothing that an Atorvastatin can't fix.*

Autoimmunity? *Steroids.*

Anxiety? *Xanax.*

Depression? *Zoloft!*

Pain? *Tylenol, ibuprofen, gabapentin. Still in pain? – so many narcotics to choose from!*

Do you see the unhealthy pattern here? What if we could approach these in a completely different manner?

Tired? *How about a day off?*

Exhausted? *How about a vacation? Maybe you are doing too much? Can a resource be provided so that you can take a much-needed break?*

Acid reflux? *Perhaps you are stressed? Is the cause of your stress worth the risk to your health?*

High blood sugar /high blood pressure /high cholesterol? *Maybe a diet change would help.*

Autoimmunity? *Perhaps staying away from some of the heavy chemicals hidden in processed foods, cosmetics, and cleaning supplies would give your immune system a well-deserved break.*

Anxious or depressed? *Perhaps your body is feeling what you have been trying to avoid with your mind. Or maybe you feel lonely, scared, grieving,* or are experiencing the aftereffects of a traumatic event that you have never been able to process. Maybe the trauma happened long ago, but for you, it never ended. Let's address the issues and provide resources that would help you heal.

Pain? *Let's find a cause and make appropriate changes.*

The first set of examples is what we currently do. That's why it should be called **sick-care**. The second set of examples is what we should do instead, to promote health and healing, and be able to call it **healthcare**.

Based on the first set, we deny ourselves all that the body might be asking for. We silence its communication pathways with drugs and then become surprised when we find ourselves in crisis, needing a hospital bed. Then, in the hospital, we are given more medications, and suffer more side effects, not only from the root cause of the problem but also from polypharmacy. If we are still able, we become angry with the system; we become angry with nurses, doctors, and other hospital staff. If we are no longer able, our family does it for us. We get upset because we haven't been cured. We get upset because we can't go on with our lives as usual.

We have been going to doctors all our lives and they always come up with new medications for us to take. So, what about when we are dying, or at the moment of death? Don't they have a cure for that too?

Death Denial

How much is too much? How do we stop?

I wish I had a clear answer for you. Based on my hospital experience, I would say we don't know how to stop. We often deny death and dying, just as, throughout our lives, we deny the body the opportunity to restore and heal.

In the ICU, we administer more and more medications, in more and more invasive ways. We insert tubes for feeding, tubes for urine drainage, stool tubes, blood tubes, and abscess tubes. If one medication doesn't work, we add another. To counteract side effects, we add a third. If that doesn't work, we deliver more medicines in drip form. Drips are medications infused continuously at a rate that is frequently being adjusted. Patients' lives are often dependent on these drips. Running out of one drip, even for a minute, can lead to cardiac arrest. The nurses must be vigilant to never run out of these life-sustaining drips, and be sure to order them from the pharmacy ahead of time.

Imagine the case of a heavily medicated patient in the ICU. Their body becomes swollen beyond recognition, and organs start failing one by one. They develop skin blisters and muscle wasting called atrophy. Fingers and toes become nonviable and black from lack of perfusion, caused by medications that cut off peripheral circulation in order to maintain perfusion to the heart. The organ battle mentioned earlier is on! Which one to choose – the heart or the kidneys? The lungs or the heart? The brain or the kidneys? What about the liver?

Despite our division into specialties and subspecialties, all the body's organs are interconnected and interdependent. Our efforts to save one often compromise the well-being of another.

Medical interventions can cause tremendous pain and have serious side effects. We use medications to ease that pain, and sedation to dull consciousness, but the side effect of these medications is dropping already-low blood pressure, causing further harm to the organs. Should we keep the patient comfortable, pain-free, and unconscious at the cost of their kidneys? To try and save the kidneys while keeping the patient pain-free, we add drips that raise blood pressure, but may further compromise the liver. Despite our efforts, the patient often ends up on dialysis. Dialysis drops the blood pressure further, so we add more medication to raise it. We start with one drip; if that doesn't help, we add another. We add a third if the blood pressure is still falling, despite the two infusions. We can keep adding, but usually after four of five of these drips, the kidneys have already failed; other organs like the liver and lungs begin to fail, and the patient dies.

If we increase our life-saving efforts but the patient does not respond favorably, the physician will speak to the family to explain what is happening and to ask them about their wishes. The family has an option to sign a Do Not Resuscitate (DNR) form or not. If the form is signed and the patient's heart stops, the patient dies.

If the document is not signed and the heart stops, cardiopulmonary resuscitation (CPR) is initiated, and the advanced cardiovascular life support (ACLS) guidelines are followed. Everyone in the ICU is trained and certified on these strict guidelines, which include a systematic way of performing chest compression, checking for a pulse, and administering emergency medications. If the patient's pulse returns, the CPR is over, and our efforts to keep them alive continue. It is common to perform CPR multiple times until the pulse does not return and the patient dies.

This whole process may happen quickly or may happen for weeks. One step forward, two steps back. Two steps forward, one step back. Just when things are turning for the better, the patient may get an infection caused by all the tubes and drains attached to their body, or they may develop a bedsore from being bed-bound and on medications that compromise blood perfusion to their skin. The families get tired, frustrated, and angry. They may start blaming themselves or the medical staff. They often feel helpless and inadequate. They have to make the most difficult decisions they can ever face, such as consenting to invasive lines or tubes, dialysis, tracheotomy, or the DNR itself.

In such times of desperation and grief, families often become vocal in their religious beliefs. They turn to God. They affirm their belief in a deity and say, "Do everything you can, please." They also say, "It's in God's hands now." I've heard both of these many times.

The Death Fighting Dilemma

What happens after death? Science has no empirical answer to this question. What we do know is that we all must die. Scary? Yes, since we don't know how, or when, or who will go first. As this is the case, how can we be ready and accept the outcome, whichever way it goes? Accepting the fact of death is all that's in our power. Could it be that by accepting death, we can become empowered? In this way, could we change the process of dying from one of distress and fear, into one of acceptance and courage?

Nothing in our culture nowadays prepares us for the fact of death. The focus of our society is to oppose aging: from anti-wrinkle cream to cosmetic surgery. Twenty-year-olds get Botox now!

When the elderly are no longer able to look after themselves, what do we do with them in our materialistic society? They simply don't fit! Their families can't take care of them, because they themselves must work. Communities don't exist much anymore, especially for those in need of help or support. Nursing homes – which after all are a business just like hospitals, despite what they advertise – often lack the proper number of caregivers.

Then when the time to die finally comes, what do we do? We panic!

In our panic, we produce so much disarray. So many resources are used to stop death; trash cans upon trash cans are filled to the top with equipment, medications, blood bags, tubes, drains, catheters, isolation gowns the works. Bags are filled with linen drenched with body fluids, like blood, stool, urine, and mucus. Our medical skills are so perfected that we can now administer up to 575 milliliters of blood a minute. That's your body's entire blood volume, replaced in approximately 8.7 minutes. Imagine transfusing this way for hours on end.

We can fight the body's decline for a very long time. Sometimes we win, sometimes we lose, but I can tell you *every time* we sure as hell put up a fight.

Cancer, a major cause of death in many societies, begins with cells that mutate and seek independence from the rest of the body. To achieve that independence, they kill the body upon which they depend.

I sometimes wonder when humanity will become aware of how cancerous and self-destructive **we** are. Will our society, including all the big corporations, politicians, and people with privilege and power, ever come to this awareness? And if or when we do, and our efforts change direction, will we still be able to turn it around? Or will our civilization need to die for the world to rebuild itself?

The Time Is Now

All too often, we realize the value of something only after we lose it.

I remember a patient complaining about the food on his tray. He had type II diabetes and his hospital diet was sugar-free. He had lost his vision, plus a couple of toes, due to his disease. He was in the ICU because he was losing perfusion (blood flow) to his leg, and the doctors were trying to surgically re-perfuse it to save his limb and avoid amputation. He asked me to shave his beard, and while I was doing so, we got into an interesting conversation.

He told me that he used to work at a candy bar factory, producing world-renowned candy bars known to us all I remember enjoying them when I was a kid. He reminisced about the days when he could see, and the beautiful things that now only existed in his memory.

He did not know, or perhaps refused to acknowledge, the impact of sugar on his declining condition. I explained it to him in the simplest of ways. I then asked him, with what he now knew, if he were to live again, would he take steps to prevent it? Would he change his lifestyle to prevent the loss of his vision and his toes? Would he try to avoid all this pain and suffering if he were given another chance at life? Would he give up sugar in exchange for his health?

He took a moment and answered decisively, "Yes, I would do it. I would rather see."

Then I told him: "How about I tell you that you will get to keep your leg if you change your diet now?"

He smiled, and never complained about his sugar-free tray again.

The time for change is always now. We can't go back in time and fix our mistakes, but we can always change the decisions we make right now, in our current situatuion, therefore preventing more from happening in the future. When we're content but someone challenges us to grow, let's pause and reflect instead of reacting with anger or dismissal—resisting change only prolongs our own suffering.

It should be obvious by now that our healthcare system is in desperate need of improvement. It is also clear that, instead of waiting for politicians and lobbyists to have a change of heart, we need to take things into our own hands. The change that we would like to see must first happen within each of us. We are the necessary change. The powers that be would have us remain in ignorance, but we mustn't let that continue.

We must make it our business to become knowledgeable. What are the things that keep us healthy and what are the things that make us sick? Only then do we start to have a choice.

I hope this book will help you change your own life and contribute to creating the healthcare system we need. Don't wait to get trapped in the sick-care system. Start practicing healthcare today.

Part 2

Reclaiming Health

Chapter 4

Through Mindfulness to Awareness

Introduction to Mindfulness and Awareness

Mindfulness is the practice of focusing attention on the present moment by observing our thoughts, emotions, bodily sensations, and environment with an open and non-judgmental mindset. Awareness is a broader concept that involves gaining a deeper understanding of ourselves and our motivations. Awareness requires the ability to step back and evaluate our thoughts, emotions, and behaviors from an impartial perspective. In essence, mindfulness is a component of awareness that encompasses various aspects of conscious perception and understanding in daily life.

How Mindfulness Connects to Health and Well-being

What do mindfulness and awareness have to do with health and well-being? Everything! They provide the antidote to stress and anxiety. Questioning their role is like doubting the importance of our mental state to our overall health.

Health is not limited to the physical body, a false concept often portrayed in our current healthcare system. Health is so much more. It's a way of life that has to be worked at. To practice health we should practice mindfulness, as well as taking care of our physical well-being.

Action and Reaction in Life

Our existence consists of actions and experiences, in particular our reactions to those experiences. Choosing not to act is still a form of reaction. Whether at home, school, or work, we're constantly reacting to everything around us, shaping our lives moment by moment.

Some actions provoke our immediate attention. For example, as a nurse in the Intensive Care Unit (ICU) of a hospital, the quicker my response, the better the chances of the patient surviving.

But it does not need to be a life-threatening situation to provoke an instant need to react. During a family gathering or interactions with children, a spouse, colleagues, friends, a difficult neighbor, or even an acquaintance, this same need can arise. Recall how quickly you may have been provoked in the past. Inaction, although an option, seems nearly impossible; our response is often so immediate that it's as if we have no choice at that moment. The person speaking may not have even finished their sentence when, in our mind, we have already formulated a reply, ready to deliver an immediate comeback.

Responsibility and 'Respond-ability'

Awareness is about creating space between action and reaction – between what happens and how we react. By practicing it, we can train ourselves to slow down time, allowing choice to arise and providing us a space in which we can respond more thoughtfully.

This ability to respond is the "respond-ability," or responsibility referred to by Sadhguru Vasudev in his book *Inner Engineering: A Yogi's Guide to Joy*.

Sadhguru Jaggi Vasudev is a prominent Indian yogi, mystic, and author. He is the founder of the Isha Foundation, a multifaceted organization dedicated to spiritual growth and well-being through yoga and spiritual practices, environmental initiatives, and social outreach programs all around the world. He explains the process thus:

> *Being fully responsible is to be fully conscious... Responsibility is a much-misunderstood term. It has been used so widely and indiscriminately that it has lost much of its inner voltage. Responsibility does not mean taking on the burdens of the world. It does not mean accepting blame for things you have done or not done. It does not mean living in a state of perpetual guilt.*

> *Responsibility simply means your ability to respond. If you decide, I am responsible, you will have the ability to respond. If you decide, I am not responsible, you will not have the ability to respond. It is as simple as that. All it requires is for you to realize that you are responsible for all that you are and all that you are not, all that may happen to you and all that may not happen to you.*[25]

Importance of Awareness in High-Stress Environments

Imagine you are a trauma nurse receiving a patient from the operating room who has suffered severe trauma, such as multiple gunshot wounds, or injuries from a motor vehicle accident. Despite tremendous efforts by the medical team, the patient's condition continues to deteriorate. The Massive Transfusion Protocol (MTP) is activated and the Rapid Infusion System (RIS) deployed a device used to infuse blood or other fluids, which can replace the patient's entire blood volume multiple times within an hour.

Or you receive a patient in the ICU with dangerously low and unstable blood pressure that instantly drops when blood transfusion and life-sustaining medications are interrupted. Sure, you have your team to back you up, but this is "your" patient and you are the one ultimately responsible for coordinating their care. They're cold, bleeding profusely onto the bed sheets, and the drainage containers are filling up fast. Every second counts; your choice of action and priorities will determine whether or not you can save their life.

How do you keep calm and make the right decisions?

Knowledge, experience, resources, and teamwork – all are required. But for me, awareness is just as necessary. An ICU nurse must stay in control during these stressful situations. By practicing awareness, I keep my stress

---

[25] Sadhguru, "Inner Engineering: A Yogi's Guide to Joy", 2016.

and anxiety levels low. I do not panic. I acknowledge my emotions without letting them overwhelm me. I stay in control.

Staying aware allows me to eliminate racing thoughts and doubts, and focus on each task. It clears mental space for analyzing options. I may feel it has taken minutes to reach a decision, but in reality, it only took a second.

That's the space of awareness, and that's how staying aware feels to me. It doesn't mean that I slow down. On the contrary, my mind slows down but my decision-making speeds up.

Awareness in Personal Relationships

The same principle applies in everyday situations. Within families, for example, heated arguments can erupt from nowhere. Between spouses or partners, hurtful things are said in a flash. Imagine your teenage child pushing your buttons to the point where you say something you regret almost immediately. The sense of release soon gives way to a feeling of guilt.

Then there is the issue of approaching difficult subjects. Your fifteen-year-old son has developed a habit of skipping class. You are concerned and emphasize the importance of junior year in shaping his future career. He dismisses your concern with a confident smile, insisting that he has 'got this' and urging you to 'chill.'

Chill! Every time you screw up and you come asking for help, you want me to chill?"

He says, "*Okay, chill bro!*"

You say you are not his bro; you are his mother. You tell him he's wasting his life and that you do so much for him. You tell him you're sick of him and of the way he talks to you.

In situations like these, what if you could take time to think and choose a better response? Instead of making your son defensive, you could make him think about the consequences of his actions. With awareness, you might say something like this:

I worry when you skip class because junior year is a crucial time in preparing for your future. But I trust you to understand that, and to make the right decisions.

This approach might make him more receptive to your concerns.

Always remember that you have control over your reactions. Of course you're worried that he won't get into a good college or get a job. You're afraid that he'll spend all his days playing video games, never move out, or be able to provide for himself. But if you take a step back from your fear and from insisting that he sees things your way, you're free to react in any way you desire. You can even have some fun with it, and to his *"chill, bro"* comment, respond:

"Well, bro, you my homie need to get your shit together, all right!"

How about that Thanksgiving dinner with the family when your entire life's purpose becomes the topic of discussion at the dinner table? When the jokes are no longer funny and the atmosphere becomes tense? All of a sudden, your loving family members are questioning your beliefs, opinions, and decisions. You are thrown off balance.

What if you could stay "aware" during such challenging situations? Create space, and give yourself the necessary time to respond thoughtfully.

Time Perception and Awareness

In this space of awareness, we perceive time differently. It may feel as if we've taken an age to process our feelings, but in fact only a few seconds have passed.

Imagine having more room through which to navigate that difficult conversation. Imagine experiencing it in slow motion, enabling you to acknowledge different feelings within yourself. You could use this time to reflect on past experiences and their outcomes, empowering you to respond according to your values and avoiding future regrets.

Imagine having that time to yourself, and no one notices you have taken it. Would it not be of benefit in your family and professional relationships, or with your friends?

Mindfulness as a Foundation for Healthy Relationships

Practicing mindfulness gives us a heightened awareness, enabling us to establish health within ourselves and in our relations to others. Having healthy relationships is a proven factor in leading a long and fulfilling life, but the relationship to and within the self is the most important of all. Once we have a healthy relationship with ourselves, we can build healthy relationships with others.

Practical Ways to Practice Mindfulness

Mindfulness requires that we pay attention. That may sound easy, but it may be quite challenging to put into practice.

There are many ways to practice paying attention. Some of the most successful ways I know are meditation, yoga, and breathing exercises. All are part of the Inner Engineering program developed by Sadhguru that offers tools for inner transformation.[26] I will explore these strategies further in **Chapter 8** under the subtitle **Spa Alternatives**.

For now, let's explore other dimensions of awareness necessary to understand all aspects of health.

---

26 Isha.sadhguru.org

Awareness of the System

Dependence on Social Systems

We cannot deny our dependence on the healthcare system. Just as we rely on legal and economic systems, our society leans heavily on healthcare. Our parents and families made great efforts to ensure our integration into these systems and much of our success is judged by how well we fit within them.

Everyone Contributes to The Healthcare System

As members of society, our involvement with the healthcare system is unavoidable. Everyone is a potential patient as, at some point in our lives, we will probably all require medical care. Even if we don't, we will still be required to shoulder the financial burden that keeps our healthcare system in place. This is the view we must take to get involved and help put in place the necessary changes to make it better.

The Reality of Trauma and Healthcare Dependency

For those who are still not convinced of their involvement, let's imagine a scenario we don't dare to imagine – trauma. What if, as a result of a traumatic car crash, you suffer brain damage that completely impairs your ability to make decisions?

It is a harsh reality that hospitalization can occur regardless of our will.

You might have led a healthy lifestyle, but you have now become subjected to intensive direct care. Furthermore, hospital treatment, including diagnostic testing and surgical interventions, will proceed regardless of your preferences.

Transformation of the System

We take our health for granted until we become sick and diseased, and typically only seek medical intervention after much of the damage has already been done. We enter the healthcare system only when we reach a point of desperation, unable to ignore debilitating symptoms any longer.

We seek medical attention and, instead of exploring the lifestyle changes that could potentially help us, we opt for medications as a quick fix.

Unity of Mind, Body, and Spirit

The current disease-oriented approach to health has proven ineffective. It is time to revamp our current system into a health-oriented model that focuses on uniting the realms of mind, body, and spirit. We need a system that considers the balance between our *"inner and outer worlds – natural, familial, communal, and metaphysical."*[27] All cultures embrace practices intended to maintain well-being, such as food, movement, social connections, rituals, healing practices, and traditions, as many experts assert.[28]

Global Interconnectedness and Environmental Impact

As a nation, we fail to recognize the unity of our mind, body, and spirit. This oversight mirrors our failure to recognize our interconnectedness with the rest of the world. By focusing solely on the well-being of our own country and consuming excessive global resources, we jeopardize the environmental and economic security of other nations. If we continue down this path, we will irredeemably damage our planet and cause immense human suffering. Our selfish actions as a nation are creating a harmful reality that, if continued, will lead to our self-destruction.

---

27 Southard et al., 2020.
28 Southard et al., 2020.

Awareness of Personal Bias

Interdependence and Collective Consequences

We are all consumers and all connected to each other. Every individual's actions contribute to a collective consequence, and our current healthcare system reflects this collective action and inaction.

Convenience and Lack of Appreciation

We have made our lives very convenient. What past generations had to devote most of their lives toward achieving, the current generation has acquired with very little effort. Life is more convenient than ever before, yet people are feeling more stressed and anxious. Technological and scientific advancements in agriculture mean that the majority of us in the first world no longer need to spend all our time producing food.

My grandparents were farmers, spending most of their lives working on the land to put food on the table. A lot of hard work went into feeding the family. Now, most of us are paid for the skills we employ at work and use the money we earn to buy whatever we want at the store. Everything is so accessible and convenient that we often fail to appreciate it.

Anxiety Caused by Overwhelming Abundance of Choice

With so much availability, we now face the challenge of making the right choice. A quick stop at the store to pick up some deodorant has turned into an ordeal, due to the overwhelming variety available. A dizzying array of different scents, colorful packaging, catchy sale pitches, and *"no harmful chemicals"* labels make you question this abundance. Are you someone who picks up three different deodorants, unable to choose the best? Or, like me, do you leave the store empty-handed, putting off the dilemma for some other day? Perhaps you reassure yourself that it's all right not to use deodorant!

Information Overload and Manipulation

If just a trip to the grocery store presents us with countless choices, to make matters worse, we're bombarded with misinformation. We are continuously manipulated by corporations seeking to maximize their profits. Unfortunately, the bigger the company, the more power they have to corrupt and extend their financial influence over educators, doctors, scientists, and even local and federal governments. Federal laws are often influenced or even drafted by corporate legal teams. Consider how long it took to write "*Smoking Kills*" on cigarette packaging, or calorie counts on restaurant menus.

Education and Misinformation

Nutritional labels can be misleading. We can't always trust the information we're given and should always be mindful of the source and its economic angle.

People often say it comes down to self-education. While I agree with that to some degree, I believe we must approach information sources with a critical eye. We are inundated with misinformation on product labels, and with data manipulation on the internet.

I highly recommend watching Jeff Orlowski's 2020 documentary *The Social Dilemma*, which portrays this problem in detail.

Advertisement Revenue Model and Internet Search Engines

It's essential to understand that search engines and internet sites like Google, Bing and Facebook are driven by an advertising revenue model. Their algorithms prioritize popular or paid content over truthful information, to maximize clicks and advertising revenue. They create an alternative commercial reality in which the consumer's best interests are not part of the equation.

Search results are personalized based on your browsing history. The more you search for a particular idea, the more likely you are to find information reinforcing that idea. The search engine will not sort through the morass of information on your behalf, picking what is true. Nor will it correct your view if you are wrong. That work is entirely up to you.

As highlighted in *The Social Dilemma*, search engines will not present everything available on the subject. Instead, they give you the content most likely to engage you further, which may include irrelevant or misleading information.

Biases in AI Systems

AI systems, including chatbots and virtual assistants, which are designed to conduct human-like conversations with users through text or voice interactions, are definitely not infallible. Although they can provide personalized responses and recommendations, they can make mistakes, misinterpret queries, and give outdated or incorrect information. They inherit biases from the data used to train them. This can perpetuate harmful stereotypes and class and racial discrimination.

While AI can be incredibly useful, it's important to think critically about the information it provides and to fact-check this against reliable sources.

Confirmation Bias and Emotional Attachments

The more deeply you go into a particular subject, the more you may inadvertently reinforce your biases. As you spend time learning about an issue, you may also feel increasingly confident speaking about it to others.

You may feel you wish to educate them.

By then, you might have developed an emotional attachment to the subject matter, increasing the possibility of confirmation bias. Confirmation Bias is the tendency to interpret new evidence as confirmation of one's existing beliefs or theories, dismissing contradictory information. Failure to recognize bias leads to the illusion of absolute knowledge; in other words, 'being right'. It fosters a feeling of superiority, causing you to judge views different from your own as inferior. Judgment breeds prejudice, and prejudice can lead to violence.

Awareness is the Key

You may argue,

Okay, I've probably been biased, but the connection to violence seems far-fetched.

But that's how the internet works. You are not the only one who has been biased. We have all been! Being biased is not the threat; it's the failure to recognize it that is dangerous.

Awareness of Self

Acknowledging Unawareness and Bias

Once we acknowledge our unawareness and bias, we can open our minds to new possibilities. We are better able to respond in a nonjudgmental way, and to perceive situations as they truly are, not only by how we perceive them. It is liberating!

Perceptions and Biases in Interactions

When I began to practice being aware of my perceptions, I started to feel unburdened from myself.

For example, upon meeting someone with a disability, we may instantly feel sorry for them. Where is this "feeling sorry" coming from? We just met this person. We know nothing about them. All we know is that they are in a wheelchair, or use a prosthesis, so our brain (just like a search engine) brings forth all sorts of information that is recorded under the heading 'disability.' Burdened with this information, which we believe to be true, different emotions are evoked within us. Our interaction is not then about the person we're meeting, but about ourselves.

Transforming Relationships Through Awareness

Being aware of self allows us to see the world and everything in it through a different set of eyes. Instead of viewing things solely in relation to ourselves, we see people as individuals with their unique experiences and histories, which are separate from our own. This has the power to transform relationships.

For instance, by becoming self-aware, I can regard my mother not just as "my mom," but as her own person, with a rich life story unknown and inaccessible to me. By removing **myself** from the mother-daughter relationship, I have gained insight into who **she** is as a person in her own right, rather than what she represents to me.

Liberation from Self-Insertion

Paradoxically, as I become more proficient in my practice of awareness and learn not to insert myself into each situation, I become more aware of my unawareness.

Let me give you an example: My beloved and I took a walk on the beach the other day. We passed some fishermen, one of whom had a friendly dog that greeted us eagerly, wagging its tail. I responded to the dog's friendly greeting and a conversation started up between the fisherman and ourselves. He reflected on his retired life, traveling to different places in his trailer – a life I could only dream of. When he complained how hard things were, I have to say I dismissed him with a sarcastic remark, perhaps something along the lines of *"Try a 16-hour shift in an ICU unit of a safety net hospital in Chicago,"* abruptly ending our conversation. The fishermen fell silent and we walked away. Unfortunately, it was only afterward that my beloved was able to reflect on the situation with me, revealing it in a different light.

What I did to that fisherman is precisely what I don't like anyone doing to me. I undermined his feelings by downplaying the significance of what he was revealing about his life situation. I made assumptions based solely on my own judgment, without considering that his life and experiences might differ greatly from my own. Because of a compulsion to react I had, without thinking, dismissed, disrespected, and diminished his feelings. It required the intervention of someone I love and respect for me to realize how inconsiderate I had been.

Reflecting on Personal Behaviors

The truth is we all do this to one another. Acknowledging this fact is the first step to changing our behavior. Once again, I'd lost an opportunity – to learn about the life of that fisherman. But I've gained awareness and learned something significant about myself. Next time I meet someone, I will ask questions and try to understand their reality, rather than jump to conclusions based on my own assumptions. It's so simple, and yet impossible to achieve without awareness.

Interoceptive Awareness:
Listening to Your Body

Practicing awareness of the body is as important as practicing awareness of the mind. Interoception is the ability to sense and perceive the internal state of one's body. It is a feedback mechanism from your internal organs to the brain and back. It involves detecting signals from organs such as the heart, lungs, stomach, and brain. Your thoughts and emotions can influence the functioning of your internal organs, just as the signals from your organs can shape your thoughts and emotions.

For example, when you are anxious your heart rate and breathing increase as digestion slows down. Conversely, becoming aware of these sensations makes you more aware of your anxiety. Regard this awareness as an opportunity. If you choose to shift your perception of the situation and consciously work to reduce your anxiety, you can influence your body's physiological responses. By calming the mind, you can automatically slow down your heartbeat and respiratory rate, allowing for better digestion and nutrient absorption.

Role of Interoception in Emotional Awareness

Interoception plays a vital role in helping understand and interpret our body's physical state. It allows us to recognize hunger, thirst or physical discomfort. Physiological responses, such as increased heart rate or changes in breathing patterns, accompany many emotions. Impaired interoception can affect both our physical and mental well-being.

Bodily Sensation and Communication

There are five basic human senses: touch, sight, hearing, smell, and taste, each producing bodily sensations like aches, tickles, feelings of pain, pleasure, warmth, and fatigue. Pain is the most compelling way in which the body communicates with the brain. However, there are other sensations that the body uses to convey information, such as sluggishness, sleepiness, nausea, dizziness, indigestion, hunger, thirst, arousal, and feelings of heat or cold.

Interpreting Pain and Sensations

Pain is well known to all of us. It can be both easy and challenging to figure it out. For example, if you bump your head, it hurts; therefore, the body's message is simple: *"Don't bump your head."*

But what if you have a headache without an injury? Then it's harder to pinpoint the source of the pain. In this case, we must be willing to observe, learn, and make necessary changes.

Think of it as a puzzle that the body presents, which we, the great detectives, are on a mission to solve. By solving the puzzle, we earn the prize of optimal health. In this scenario, a great detective wouldn't simply take a pill to mask the pain; that would be tampering with the evidence, wouldn't it?

First off, our detective would start making enquiries:

"When did your headache first occur?"

"Is it related to anything you ate or did the day before the symptom arose?"

With the data now collected, we become scientists. We conduct experiments. We start manipulating different variables, perhaps limiting our diet to gluten-free or sugar-free for a while, to see if the headaches will go away.

The same fieldwork applies to all the sensations which our body uses to communicate with us. It is the investigative work which doctors do – or should be doing. The difference is that we have the upper hand because it is our body, not theirs. The decision on what to do with the information we have gathered is up to us. Yes, they have the great resources of years of training and education, but the final decision should be ours, unless an emergency or trauma occurs, which I will discuss further in the book.

Challenges of Ignoring Body Signals

Unfortunately, we often ignore the messages, silence the symptoms with medications, and push our bodies to the point of no return. We find excuses not to take the appropriate action, and fail to respond to our body with the respect it deserves. We abuse it as if it were an entity separate from ourselves, not recognizing that our life and all it encompasses cannot exist without it.

We behave rather like cancer cells. Just as they build their rebellious microsystem in an attempt to take us over, we try to shape our own reality. Like cancer cells, we lack awareness of how our actions harm. We fail to understand that in succeeding with our made-up reality, we will no longer be able to exist, since we have destroyed the structure of this existence which is our body.

Unawareness

The Illusion of Health Expertise

Chances are you have tried to be proactive and prevent disease. Perhaps you work a demanding job just to secure insurance and be able to pay for your doctor's visits. You take all your medications as prescribed and never miss any appointments. You think that you have done everything necessary to stay healthy.

I hate to break it to you, but the doctors you seek help from are part of the same culture as the rest of us. Even though they have studied the body and undergone years of rigorous medical training, they too fall prey to bias and unawareness. They often learn unhealthy ways of coping with their demanding work. Many push their own bodies through exhaustion and lack of sleep, enduring long shifts or studying intensively for exams. They too can be biased or swayed in their practice by pharmaceutical companies and other corporate interests. After all, medical schools are often the target of financial influence.

Symptom Masking and Medication Culture

Too often we seek medical expertise only when we don't feel well. We leave the doctor's office with a new prescription that takes away the uncomfortable symptom, rather than the doctor genuinely looking to find what is causing that symptom. Pain medication masks symptoms and silences the body's way of communicating deeper problems of imbalance that need addressing.

I recognize the important role prescription medications play in saving lives, and how important it is to adhere to treatment plans once a disease is diagnosed. However, I want to stress the value of making lifestyle changes to prevent diseases before they occur.

Challenges and Solutions

Even when the doctor orders blood tests and tries to do a workup to find the cause of our symptoms, they are constrained by our health insurance company and what services it will cover. Our current level of understanding of the complexities and interdependencies within the human body is decades ahead of our current standard operating procedures and protocols.

There are many valuable tests that insurance providers will not cover. The ones currently used will only show a disease after many years of being undetected, and often reveal it only in its advanced stages. The standard blood workup – complete blood count (CBC), basic metabolic panel (BMP), or even complete metabolic panel (CMP) – even though they are useful in a hospital setting, are significantly outdated when used at a doctor's office for healthy individuals seeking preventative care.

Our bodies are brilliant and far more intricate than our minds can comprehend. They consist of thousands of backup mechanisms which keep compensating for deficiencies, making the test results appear within the norm until all of our body's resources are depleted.

Do you want to wait that long? I don't. I don't think any of us do, yet that is precisely what is happening.

Luckily, new clinics are emerging where medical practitioners reject the outdated, insurance-driven approach to medicine. It is time for insurance companies to reevaluate their practices and stop profiting from the sick.

Transformation to Health-Oriented Care

Facing the reality of our healthcare system can be depressing. We may feel helpless because of our inability to change what the doctors are doing or what the insurance companies pay for. It's true that as a single individual, we can't enact much change.

But what if we team up? What if we become more aware of the problem and what we can do about it, and spread that awareness to others? We then become a team, and our collective decisions carry a significant impact. If we change the demand, we influence the supply. There is strength in numbers. Every one of us counts!

We become knowledgeable and conscious consumers who buy with awareness and not out of compulsion. We become empowered patients who focus on health rather than disease. By choosing to live a healthy lifestyle and listening to our bodies, we take control of our well-being. We stop repressing symptoms and instead acknowledge them, allowing us to get to the root of the problem. We allow healing to take place.

The Takeaways:

- Practice awareness every chance you get by noticing your thoughts without engaging in them.

  When you wake up, before you even open your eyes, ask yourself what is the first thing you are thinking.

  Before you fall asleep, what is your last thought of the day?

  When you're getting ready for work?

  When you're driving?

- Practice stillness every day.

  For at least 10 minutes a day, sit down in silence and focus on what your mind is doing.

  Is your mind busy planning the next thing you will be doing?

  Are you planning the day ahead?

  Are you getting excited about a project you want to take on?

  Are you worried, stressed, or scared as a result of the thoughts running through your head?

- Without any judgement just observe and notice.

Chapter 5

Creating Health Inside and Out

> Eastern medicinal systems—including Ayurveda and Siddha—have always been based on the perception that no two human beings are alike. The way the elements function in one person is not how they function in another. This makes them a unique designer system of medicine that is hard to standardize. The doctor prescribes differently for each person, because the treatment is based not on the ailment but on the individual's constitution. Five different people with the same symptoms will be treated differently. A deep understanding of the elements underlies this.[29]
>
> Sadhguru

Wisdom can be found in the many various ways medicine is practiced throughout the world. There is so much to learn from all of them. If we acknowledge only the Western route and disregard all others, we deprive ourselves of opportunities to learn less invasive, and often less expensive, ways of treatment. Alternative medicine places great emphasis on maintaining balance and preventing disease from happening.

Have you heard the old parable about a scientist who spent years trying to climb a certain mountain? He is convinced, after all his efforts, that he will be the first to reach that uncharted peak and obtain the enlightenment he seeks, only to find, on arriving at the summit, that an enlightened guru is already sitting there. This story signifies that science is only just starting to discover what wise people have known for generations.

We often find that new advances in science and technology confirm the logic behind ancient medicinal practices. As our understanding develops, we are beginning to realize how individual differences among people significantly influence how they respond to medical treatments. An individualized approach is essential for effective healing. This principle

---

29 Sadhguru, 2021.

has been paramount in Eastern medicine since long ago. David Sinclair in his book, *Why We Age and Why We Don't Have To*,[30] wonders if a day might come when a patient's hospital treatment will begin by printing their blueprint – in other words, their genetic code, and their microbiome (the community of microorganisms that live in the human body) – in order to choose treatment specific to their physiology. Unfortunately, we are not there yet. For now, Western medicine continues to treat the disease, not the individual. To reclaim our health, we must realize that there should be no one-size-fits-all approach. We are all different, with unique genetics, biochemistry, and microbiomes; what works for one person may not work for another.

New scientific studies show a correlation between beliefs and outcomes. The best example of this is the placebo effect, in which a person experiences an improvement in their condition or symptoms due to the power of suggestion, rather than the direct effect of a specific medical treatment. Scientific studies of this phenomenon, such as that of Newman in his article "The Placebo Effect," admit that:

> Even inactive treatment has repeatedly demonstrated a measurable, positive health response... At one time, placebos were only used in experiments as a control. However, due to their ability to make changes to the body, they have now been studied extensively as a treatment in their own right.[31]

So next time you hear about some weird home remedy, refrain from judgment. What works for one person might not work for you, but this does not invalidate it. A person more inclined to faith may respond to a simple treatment, whereas one less inclined may require something more complex. Our attitude may determine the outcome of our treatment.

---

30 Sinclair, D. A., & LaPlante, M., 2019.
31 Newman, 2017.

In his book *You Are the Placebo: Making Your Mind Matter*,[32] Dr. Joe Dispenza examines how the placebo effect works by drawing on various scientific fields like neuroscience, psychology and physics. He presents documented cases where people overcome serious illnesses like cancer, heart disease, and Parkinson's disease simply by believing in a placebo treatment. Conversely, he also discusses instances where people became ill or even died after being victims of a voodoo curse or being misdiagnosed with a fatal condition, illustrating the powerful mind-body connection.

Since embracing our uniqueness and diversity is the key to health and happiness, it is not for me to make a definitive list of what you, my reader, must do to stay healthy. Only you can make that list. However, this book contains many suggestions that might be useful and that I hope will encourage and empower you in the process of reclaiming your health.

Simplify

Has a visit to the doctor become overly complicated? Scientific medicine has become so complex that, even though our doctor speaks the same language, it feels as if we need a translator during our visits. People leave the doctor's office, clinging to the bits of information they can recognize, unable to make sense of the rest. This gives us the feeling that we aren't competent to make our own health decisions and that we must let somebody else, like a doctor, make them for us. If we want healthcare to change, we must change from being passive to becoming active participants.

So – Simplify! Ask questions!

If you still don't understand, ask more questions. Then, if you still can't make sense of what you have been told, ask for resources that would help you to understand. Don't give up! This is your body, your health. When you give up trying to understand the issues, you become a passive onlooker. *You* are your own best advocate. No one knows you better than you know yourself. (If your spouse says otherwise, you fooled them well!) No one

---

32   Dispenza, J., 2014.

is affected by your health, or lack of it, more than *you* are. You *are* your health. Or, as the saying goes: *Your health is your wealth*. Therefore, you must protect it.

We also need an interpreter at grocery stores. Try reading the ingredient list on the products you buy – I presume even chemists might have a hard time! Most of us know that too much sugar is unhealthy. But in the ingredient list, sugar is now disguised under many different names, such as dextrose, glucose, sucrose, maltodextrin, and the like. This is done to trick you into buying the product. Food companies have always known that people like sweet-tasting products. They also realize that the public these days is more aware of how unhealthy sugar is. They now attempt to manipulate us by hiding it behind disguised ingredients. But these sugar substitutes and artificial flavorings are also unhealthy – avoid ingredients such as sucralose, aspartame, Splenda, and NutraSweet.

We consumers easily forget how we are being fooled. Your grandma would not use artificial coloring, like yellow 5, in her hot pepper preserves to make them look more attractive, compromising her family's health. But the food companies we encounter at our local stores think nothing of doing so. They don't care that an additive might be cancerous, as long as they have beaten their competition and can enhance their profits. Keep in mind that you support their businesses, and what they do or don't do, each time you choose their product.

Are you feeling stressed making these "simple" decisions and understanding their impact on your health – and on the rest of the world? I know I was, but things are actually a lot simpler than they're made out to be. Don't be fooled! Make a rule that, if a product contains something you can't pronounce or don't know what it is, you won't buy it. No matter how "sugar-free" the label claims the product to be, if it tastes sweet then it's got some form of sugar in it – or even worse, an unhealthy substitute.

In the same way, as you simplify your decisions about the food you buy, I would like to encourage you to simplify other areas of your life. Mathematicians, when faced with a complex mathematical problem, are taught to solve it by first simplifying it. We need to teach ourselves to simplify our life, to experience it fully.

We can easily become sidetracked by possessions and things. By clinging to possessions, we miss the point. Things are just tools that, if used wisely, can help in the process of understanding what life is truly about. The essence of your life is you, not your things. Unlock the door of understanding by simplifying.

Let me try to put it in perspective by sharing a story from my own life.

My older brother was good at math. Not only was he good at math, but he was also good at listening and paying attention, which made him successful at school and less problematic at home. Even though I aspired to be like him, I was not. School was boring to me. Life itself, people, and adventure held my passion.

Unlike other subjects at school, which were just plain boring, I developed a fear of math which is still with me today. Nowadays I'm more aware of it. Perhaps this fear of math is due to the trauma I felt back in school in Poland. Teachers then would often pick a random name from all the students, make that child stand in front of the class at the blackboard, and ask them to solve a mathematical equation or answer other math questions from a previous lecture.

For a child like myself, who spent most of my after-school time exploring the world around me instead of studying, it was a humiliating experience. Not only was it embarrassing to not know the answers and be stared at by the entire class, but the teachers would use this opportunity to shame me with comments like, *"You are nothing like your brother!"* or *"I guess intelligence doesn't run in the family."*

On one occasion, I had a feeling my name was going to be called. I knew I wouldn't be able to solve the equation we had been given. In an effort to save myself from humiliation, I learned the answer by heart.

Sure enough, my name reverberated throughout the classroom, loud and clear. I was filled with a mixture of fear and excitement, for I had meticulously memorized the equation the teacher wanted me to solve. I began writing, confident in my preparation. The teacher and the rest of the class fell silent, watching intently as I worked. I continued through to the end, but just as I was about to reach my triumphant conclusion, the teacher interjected, *"Yes, good, but can you simplify it?"*

"What does she mean, simplify?" I thought to myself in panic. "If she finds out I don't understand any of it, and that I memorized the entire thing, I'm ruined!" My heart pounding, I stood there, completely puzzled.

The teacher came up to the board, crossing out some of the numbers I had written, and said, *"Yes, simplify it. You see, here and here."* Then she said, *"Perfect. Sit down."*

I was so relieved that she had not found me out.

And – an incredible thing! – after all the stress had passed, when I looked at that darn equation again, I realized that it was super simple.

All of us can tell a story like this. Often, it gets repeated throughout our lives. Not only do we adopt the opinions of others about ourselves and make them our reality, but we also constantly compare ourselves with others.

For example:

> *"Look at the neighbors' new car. It looks so nice, why can't we have a new car like that?"*
>
> *"Maybe we can get a better one."*
>
> *"How about getting a bigger house than they have?"*

"What about getting a better-paying job than them?"

"How come their kids are so well-behaved? Why can't ours be more like theirs?"

... and so on.

What about being happy instead, appreciating what we have? What about being genuinely happy for ourselves, our neighbors, friends, bosses, coworkers, and everyone else we meet, without making comparisons? Having lots of things may be an indicator of good credit or financial stability, which allows for more comfortable living, but it is not an indicator of happiness. Happiness is entirely up to ourselves, whatever our situation may be.

The stress we endure is often self-created. Until we realize this fact, we can't deal with it. Of course, some of this stress is beyond our control, but much of it is not. Once we realize that our inability to see different options and our constantly comparing ourselves to others causes unnecessary stress, we can begin to live our own lives.

Minimize

It is a myth that the more we have, the happier we become. There is a narrative that makes us believe that if we work hard enough, we can do what we want, eat what we like, and buy whatever we desire. And that since we work so hard, we should feel entitled to all this. But this myth is fed to us only so that others can profit from the way we live; others who aren't concerned with the happiness that we are being encouraged to pursue. We ought to realize this.

The system we currently suffer is built on consumerism. Consumerism often leads us into debt. The whole myth is a lie, and our debt accumulation is a trap. The more debt we accumulate, the more trapped we become. It is nearly impossible not to. Take college education, for example – one of the most expensive traps of this system. Some debt we can't escape, but some we can, if we become more cautious about how we live.

I would encourage you to beware of getting lost in material things. Don't live for your items; use them as tools to live an adventurous and fulfilling life. You probably do not need many – just a few would do. No need to complicate things. Simplify and minimize instead.

There is so much pressure exerted on us, even as children, to keep up with societal standards. If our parents are feeling this pressure, then it will also get passed on to us. First, it's all the developmental milestones. Second, it's doing well in school and all the subjects. Third, it's to be liked and accepted by everyone. Fourth, it's to be physically fit and look good. Fifth, it's all the extracurricular activities. As we grow up it might be money, status, travel, social media, family – and the cycle begins again.

By the time we become adults, we are so used to the pressure exerted on us that we continue it by exerting pressure on ourselves. We don't need our parents to do it for us. By the time we become parents ourselves, we don't even realize we are doing it to our children. Perfect grades, perfect score, perfect job, perfect vacation, perfect home, perfect wedding, perfect spouse, perfect child… All this pressure is mentally exhausting. And for what? To achieve something that doesn't exist? Is it worth it?

The problem is that most of us forget how to dream. When asked what we would like to do, often we don't know. We might feel agitated by the question. When we completely lose touch with ourselves, consumed by our responsibilities, we're doing exactly what I did that day in class: memorizing the equation. We memorize a certain routine and re-enact each day the same way. Because it is familiar, it gives a false sense of safety. Instead of solving the problem to find the correct answer, we get by. Memorizing might get us through life as it got me through the class, but in doing so, we miss life's essence.

Let us look at the equation of life in a different way. Minimize the pressure. First, write everything down. Ask yourself why each thing or action you hold onto is important. Write them out to discover which ones require your utmost energy and effort. Then allow yourself to imagine your life without them.

Imagine living your life without that mortgage payment, which takes such a massive chunk of your salary—a life without all this debt continually stressing you out, making you work crazy hours. How would it be to **not** spend all your time driving your children to their after-school activities? How would it feel to have time for your family, for yourself, and for everything you would love to do? Allow yourself to perceive your life differently, free from your current constraints, free from pressure. Allow yourself to dream! Get in touch with that inner essence, covered beneath all those layers of perceived responsibility. Then, just like in math, simplify everything and cross out those steps you now think are unnecessary.

It takes crossing out to simplify and minimize the equation. Solving our problems is not about adding more. Some things are not worth the precious time. Do we really need a better car, a bigger house, or different furniture to feel happy? Is the job promotion going to do it for us? The busier we get, the less time we have for reflection. The more stuff we own, the more it requires our attention. Once we have too much, we can't find half of what we need, anyway.

It is easy to get busy and accumulate more and more things, but it is difficult to slow down and get rid of them responsibly. Next time you're shopping, think not twice, but three, four, five times, about each item; do you really need it?

The same goes for taking action. Next time you are presented with an opportunity, ask yourself if it is something you will enjoy doing or will it satisfy some of that unhealthy pressure. Is it what you truly want to do or is it something you learned you should do?

Changing our attitudes impacts our children and our families. Our joy and fulfillment will spread to them. By setting an example, we'll help them to see that doing or having less gives us the ability to be free to do much more in life. Arresting consumerism one person at a time will have a tremendous impact on this planet, which we depend on for life. We all make up the system that is harming it, so it is up to each of us to stop this harm.

Recognize

Simplifying and minimizing takes time. It took me about five years to start reaping the benefits of having less, so be sure to give yourself time. Giving away some of your possessions may make you feel uncomfortable at first. It might even make you feel sad or nostalgic. You might not be able to let go of certain things just yet. But, as you keep giving things away, you will start feeling lighter and lighter in yourself. And as you start having less, you will have more time for the things that matter, and for yourself.

Having more time and getting in touch with yourself after a long period might be scary. Some people have not been able to do this for as long as they can remember. They might have longed to have more time for themselves, but not know what to do with it when they get it.

For example, for those of us who have children, they change our lives completely. The moment they are born—actually, more like at the start of conception—they take over our lives, like it was always theirs to begin with. Our life revolves around them. Then they grow up and give it back to us 20 years later. Moreover, we'd better not interfere with *their* life when they are at that age! And so, we feel alone, left to ourselves within the empty nest. The empty nest does not feel to us like an opportunity, more like a heartbreak. It is as if, when our children left home, they took our life with them.

Of course, our children leaving home is just one example of the empty nest feeling. It could be caused by losing something else of value. It might be the loss of a job, the loss of an investment, a house, a loved one, or even some of our cherished possessions. That's right: minimizing and making our nest a bit more spacious may evoke the same feelings of loss.

Recognize these feelings. Examine them. Allow yourself to feel without judgment, without the "I should" or "I shouldn't." Listen to your thoughts.

Recognize the mental noise inside your head. Recognize your perception of the situation.

You might be wondering what this has to do with health. It has everything to do with it. A lot of the denial that happens inside us, finds expression outside of us. By accepting ourselves, we prevent disease. Just as our stomach is responsible for digesting food and providing the body with needed nutrients, so too are our thoughts responsible for digesting our feelings and emotions and providing our mental state with peace and acceptance. If we don't start creating health on the inside, the outside will never manifest it.

There are many resources and methods that can assist us with this 'mental digestion'. One of the most well-known and talked about, but surprisingly difficult to start practicing, is meditation. How hard can it be to sit still in silence? For those of you that have tried, you probably already know: it can feel impossible. Despite hearing and reading about all the benefits of meditation, we often simply cannot get ourselves to do it. I struggled with it myself, until I learned about the Inner Engineering program by Sadhguru.[33]

There are many ways to learn Inner Engineering practices. Courses are offered both in person, as well as online, and in all major U.S. cities as well as the rest of the world.

For me, it all started with a four-day retreat, held at the Isha Yoga Center in Tennessee. After the retreat, the daily practices quickly became part of my life and enhanced it in ways I didn't know were possible. Maybe you, too, can look up Inner Engineering online, or Dr. Joe Dispenza's retreats and meditation, or something similar, and find a method that works for you.

Avoid allowing things to pile up until they are overwhelming. Avoiding unnecessary stress is one of the best ways of preventing disease, and leads to a happy and fulfilling life. It allows us to live in harmony with ourselves.

---

33   Sadhguru mentioned earlier.

Blame Is No Gain

As you start to become mentally attuned, you might discover some deep psychological wounds that have never truly healed. You might come to realize that many of your actions or decisions are the result of previous trauma in your life. If that is the case, acknowledge all these experiences. Let them surface. Don't push them aside. Give yourself much-needed time to heal. No matter how trivial you think your troubles have been, they need an outlet.

Realization is itself an outlet. Realization may bring many overdue tears, anger, and a strong temptation to apportion blame:

> "He did this to me."
>
> "I would've been so happy if it weren't for her."
>
> "I would've done so much with my life had it been different."
>
> "It's his fault."
>
> "It's her fault."

Does this sound familiar? We have all done it and most still do it.

The problem with blame is that it robs us of our ability to respond. If it is *their* fault, it is *their* responsibility. *They* should do something about it. But since the decisions of others are beyond our control, empowerment lies solely with ourselves. Blame is a trap. By blaming others, we enslave ourselves. Yes, they might have done this to us, or perhaps they still keep doing it. The question is, what are *we* going to do about it? How do *we* respond? We should take responsibility.

How should we apply this to the problems of the healthcare system? The first two chapters of this book are concerned with how the healthcare system evolved into the one we have today. I discussed how the wealthy and privileged, in their positions of power, made decisions, and the consequences of those decisions on our healthcare today. The wealthy and privileged have had a huge impact. We might not like all the results of their choices, but if we start blaming them, or the system they helped create, we become powerless. We lose sight of our own ability to respond to our present situation, believing that since *others* have created it, there is nothing *we* can do.

Although we may blame big business, hospital management, education, the system – whatever – we have to take account of the situation as it is and concentrate our powers on moving forward. We should use all available resources to educate ourselves about health and disease. We should seek alternative ways of treating ourselves, become conscious consumers, volunteer at hospitals all these things. We need to take responsibility, become empowered – change is up to us!

Rediscovering Joy

Imagine now that you have done all this background work. You have set the stage for health and happiness. The rest of the journey will bring you great fulfillment, now that your nest is a bit emptier and there is some space. There is potential. The whole cosmos came into being out of nothing. It's time to sit back, relax, and enjoy this new space.

Breathe it all in, feeling no constraints, and have some fun with whatever new comes your way.

Too often, as we grow older and become responsible adults, we forget how to have fun. Instead, we grow weary, stressed, somber. We drink alcohol, or take drugs, to help change our mood. It's time to discover what fun and genuine joy feels like, without toxic substances. Explore! Try new things!

We all know exercise and physical activity are beneficial to our health. We hear about it all the time. So much so, that just the word "exercise" may make us cringe, bringing out a feeling of guilt that we should be doing more. But this in turn takes the fun out of exercise. Think about it. If you

CREATING HEALTH INSIDE AND OUT

were told that joy is beneficial to your health, like I am trying to tell you, you might already be turning fun into a chore, which creates the exact opposite effect.

Don't create more responsibilities, pick up more chores, or feel more guilt. Remember to simplify, not complicate. Accept situations that you can't control and make the best out of the ones you can. Let yourself be. Appreciate yourself. So what if you haven't had the time to go to the gym? Perhaps instead, put music on and dance away all the craziness that might be going on in your head. For those who are able, dancing can raise your heart rate above 150 beats per minute, and what an excellent alternative it is. It won't feel like exercise, just pure fun, leaving you feeling joyful afterwards.

There are many different alternatives. Stay open-minded. Move that lifeless body of yours any way you feel, and watch it come alive. Maybe the crazier you get, the more fun it will be.

"Welcome to Earth" is a series of episodes from National Geographic that I have enjoyed.[34] Actor Will Smith joins explorers of the world on some of their most extreme adventures. Each time he does something new, he must face the fear within himself. He discovers that facing and overcoming fear brings a great sense of accomplishment and fulfillment at the end of the journey.

How do we get past the fear and apathy that we might be feeling when trying to exit our comfort zone? We must cultivate a childlike curiosity and that feeling of being alive. When that feeling sparks into being, go for it! Don't let fear and doubt stop you.

You may have forgotten what childlike curiosity feels like. Give yourself time and pay attention to your feelings. A glimpse of wonder may come, and you may automatically try to ignore it. Notice as you do that. Bring it back and listen to it. What evoked the feeling of excitement? If it's drinking, drugs, or casual sex, I urge you to dig much deeper than that. You

---

[34] National Geographic. (2021). *Welcome to Earth* [TV series]. Disney+.

may need to refrain from those to reconnect with that lost part of yourself, that childlike curiosity and excitement. These are key to becoming totally involved in whatever activity you choose. Being fully engaged makes you lose yourself to the point of blissfulness.

For instance, when you cook, cook like a child who has never done it before. Taste, smell, and listen, as if it is your first time. Apply this principle every time you get a chance, and see how your life is transformed.

The Takeaways:

- Whenever you are tempted to buy, ask yourself, do I want it or do I need it? Limit yourself to buying the things you want only on special occasions.
- Buy used, it's great for our planet.
- Gift others with your unwanted things, rather than tossing them away.
- Research the companies you are gifting with your unwanted things to make sure they are giving back to the community.
- Make a rule to not buy more without finishing the products you already have. Apply this rule to foods and cosmetics. If you bought something but no longer want it, deal with it before buying another one.
- If you like to explore garage sales and markets, do so with admiration for the things you see, without the urge to buy compulsively. You can still have fun and be grateful for all the wonderful things, without possessing them.

Declutter your home responsibly. Pay attention to every little thing you've accumulated over the years. Decide if it can be useful to others before throwing it away. This will make you a much more conscious consumer.

Chapter 6

Listening to the Body's Needs

What I mean by listening to the body's needs is embracing and living in harmony with our body. Rather than suppressing bodily reactions through drugs or unhealthy habits, why not look at them as a guide? Instead of exerting control, let's be humble and be guided by our body's remarkable abilities; see the body as the miraculous vessel of life that it is – something to be protected, appreciated and celebrated, not abused or criticized. Let's appreciate its capabilities, instead of worrying about any perceived flaws that need "fixing." Why try to fix what isn't broken? Let's just not break it! Gratitude leads to graceful aging, with each life lesson engraved on our faces. Wisdom does not need plastic surgery.

To each of our actions there is a bodily reaction. It can be a simple process: we drink water—we need to use the washroom afterward. Or it can be complex: we suffer a traumatic accident; in which case many different healing processes are required for our survival. The body responds and adjusts to everything we do and to everything that happens to us. These actions/reactions are automatic, and we are scarcely aware of them taking place. We are unaware, for instance, of the release of insulin after eating.

It is often more convenient for us to disregard our bodily reactions and ignore their subtle messages.

For example:

You might have eaten something that your body is working hard to digest and, as a result, you become sleepy. Because you are at work, you counteract the sleepiness by drinking coffee. Maybe you are often sleepy, so drinking coffee becomes your routine method of staying awake. However, the effects of the caffeine mask the true cause of your sleepiness: the food you are eating.

What if, in addition to eating unhealthy food, you stay up late during the weekend to catch up on all your favorite shows, as you don't have to wake up early for work? Because the shows keep you engaged, you don't feel sleepy or tired while watching them. When the work week starts, however, you find yourself feeling drained, and one cup of coffee is not enough.

Once this pattern becomes established, and you start drinking three or more cups a day, you will be putting your body in a state of inflammation, where disease is almost inevitable.

We must take these subtle messages on board to forestall illness. By listening to the body, we give ourselves a chance of preventing disease. Taking note of the consequences of our actions allows us to correct harmful behaviors. Often, we rebel against healthy behaviors, as if we were children rebelling against our parents. In the same way children fail to appreciate their parents' efforts to keep them safe, we fail to appreciate the persistent efforts our cells make to keep us in optimal health. Such unawareness can result in our self-destruction. Our own actions are so damaging that our cells can no longer compensate for our thoughtless behavior toward ourselves.

No magic pill can bring our health back after the damage has been done. Medications often help manage a disease, but are not the cure for it. The notion of a "magic pill" that can instantly restore health is a myth perpetuated by the pharmaceutical industry, which profits from selling treatments rather than cures.

Instead of looking for a bottle of pills, we should reflect on our lifestyle. What changes are required to bring beneficial results? Far more than we realize, the state of our health is a reflection of all the actions and decisions we make. Eating the right foods is crucial in this regard. What we put into our body plays a vital part in maximizing its potential. We will feel better if we eat better. The decision is ours.

Conscious Consumers

I am grateful for all the nutritious and healthy produce grown worldwide, which I can now enjoy just by shopping at my local grocery store. The aisles are neatly stocked with all manner of fruits and vegetables; but nothing comes without a price. I am fully aware of the struggles and hardships that are involved in their production.

When I was a child, this variety of exotic fruits and vegetables was not as readily available. In the summer especially, instead of shopping for groceries at one of our city's stores, we would spend the weekend at our grandparents' farm about two hours away from Krakow. We would return home with the car packed full to the brim of in-season fruits and vegetables. Everything was so ripe and delicious. The reason for this was that my grandparents grew their produce each year from their own seed, so its nutritional value was preserved through the process of reseeding. None of their seed was genetically modified, but had been passed down through generations of crops.

Unfortunately, in the United States, seeds are now patented. When farmers purchase a patented seed, they sign an agreement that they will not save or replant seeds produced from those they buy.[35] The seeds they buy each year are genetically modified; one major reason for this is to withstand the chemical *glyphosate*. Glyphosate is the main ingredient of the weedkiller *Roundup*.

Around 94 percent of soybean crops and 90 percent of cotton and corn grown in the United States now comes from genetically altered seeds. This results in reduced cost and increased crop yields but, according to the International Agency for Research on Cancer, glyphosate is a probable cause of the disease. Because of this, at the present time (2024), there are thousands of lawsuits ongoing against Bayer, the makers of *Roundup*.

Also, we should not overlook the pernicious effect that federal agricultural subsidies are having on the nation's health, and on the farmers themselves. My heart goes out to those no longer able to hold on to their family farms, as a direct result of these subsidies. As Tara O'Neill Hayes and Katerina Kerska from the American Action Forum (AAF) write:

---

35 Hopkins, 2013.

> *The U.S. government heavily influences what farmers grow and consumers eat through various policies to subsidize the production of certain crops. The most highly subsidized crops particularly corn, wheat, and soy are highly prevalent in our food supply and consumed at rates well above recommendations, especially in highly processed foods.*"[36]

Besides having to combat the effects of ever-increasing industrialization, farmers also experience firsthand what is happening to our climate. Declining soil quality and harsh weather conditions, with drought and floods posing a severe threat to their crops, are making their task ever harder.

We must reverse the severe damage that has already been done. To do this, we must return to sustainable agriculture and regenerative systems of food production. Sustainable agriculture aims to sustain the land and economy by working with natural processes rather than against them. Regenerative agriculture is a way of farming that aims to improve the environment. It increases biodiversity, enriches soil health, protects water sources and enhances natural ecosystem processes.

An important aspect of regenerative agriculture is capturing and storing carbon in the soil, which helps reduce the amount of carbon dioxide in the atmosphere. Instead of just slowing down the depletion of resources, its goal is to restore land, boost productivity, and create a better environment through sustainable farming methods.

Farmers all around the world are fighting to save their way of life in the teeth of corporate agri-industry. One way we can be part of the necessary change is to become an 'Earth Body' at consciousplanet.org and join the "Save Soil" movement. Changes must take place at the legislative level, but

---

36   O'Neill Hayes et al., 2021.

for this to happen, activists like Sadhguru, and like-minded people from all over the world, need our support.

Since most of us don't grow our own food anymore, we must inform ourselves about its source. Is it being produced sustainably?

However trivial our decisions about the products we buy and the food we eat might seem, they have a profound impact on the farmers who supply it. Just as we must care for our caregivers, we must start caring for our farmers. Without their knowledge and skills, our urban lives would not be possible. As they are the source, they are placed at the bottom of the supply chain in our market economy. Manufacturers, distributors, and retailers consume large portions of the pie, leaving only crumbs for the suppliers.

Applied Science of Nutrition

A nursing degree is considered a degree in applied science. However, beyond my use of science in an acute care setting, fighting life-threatening diseases with pharmaceuticals, I felt myself inept in other aspects of health — in particular, disease prevention. Because I was a nurse, friends and family members would ask me simple questions about their diet and lifestyle, which I couldn't answer. Perplexed, I didn't know how to explain to them that modern hospital nursing is not what they think. But I wanted my nursing practice to be everything they thought it was. I decided to take matters into my own hands and look for knowledge beyond my clinical nursing education.

My current knowledge of nutrition does not come from nursing school or nursing practice. My interest was fired by programs such as "The Functional Nutrition Lab," run by Andrea Nakayama, with all the wonderful resources she provides. I signed up for a year-long "Full Body Systems" training with Andrea.

It was everything I hoped it would be and, for the first time, I felt as if I could apply my knowledge outside the hospital setting. I was excited about everything I was learning and correcting omissions in my clinical practice I had never noticed before. Conversations with some of the physicians at work around these topics made me realize that they are often trapped in the same way I was. We're full of scientific and clinical knowledge that serves little purpose outside the hospital walls.

Thanks to Andrea Nakayama and her work, a whole new world has opened up for me that I couldn't keep to myself, and which has inspired me to write this book.

One of many interviewees included in Andrea's program is Dr Wahls who, in the course of extensive research in nutrition and autoimmunity, has precisely analyzed the nutritional contents of different foods. Thanks to this research, we know that instead of supplements and pills we just need to eat whole foods that are nutritious. Her groundbreaking work on managing multiple sclerosis has given back quality of life to many who are suffering from the disease.

If you suffer from autoimmune disorders and are curious to learn more, I recommend her incredible book, *The Wahls Protocol: A Radical New Way to Treat All Chronic Autoimmune Conditions Using Paleo Principle.* In it, Dr. Wahls writes:

Some 70 to 95 percent of the risk of developing autoimmune problems, obesity, heart disease, and mental health problems comes from the environment. "Environment" means what you eat, what you drink, what you breathe in, what you bathe in, how you move, and even how you think and interact with people. What really matters is how your genes interact with the accumulation of your choices. This is what will determine whether you have good health or develop a chronic disease. The key is to know how to shift the odds toward achieving the most optimal health, given the genes

> that you were born with, by making your internal environment -your cellular environment- as favorable as possible."[37]

I am grateful to have become acquainted with other passionate physicians, practitioners and individuals who have experienced, and often suffered, the consequences of the disease-oriented sick care practiced in Western medicine. They have transformed their negative experience into a gift that they are now sharing with the rest of us, giving us all a chance at health.

Fake Food

Food is fuel for the body. There are many different types of foods on which our bodies can run, just as there are different types of fuels. The body's performance depends on the quality of that fuel.

It is essential to nourish the body and not to eat merely to stave off hunger.

New scientific discoveries have proved not eating to be beneficial to our health. Not eating allows the body to focus on something other than digestion, giving it an opportunity to heal itself. These new discoveries have refocused attention on the ancient practice of fasting. Many ways of fasting are becoming popular: it turns out that temporary hunger is good for us. This should not be confused with the hunger that leads to starvation, sadly prevalent in parts of the world today. But refraining from food voluntarily can promote health, support cellular repair and even slow down aging.

To feed an ever-growing population, the food industry relies on mass production of cheap flour, sugar, soy and high fructose corn syrup-filled foods that appeal to our taste buds. Rather than alleviating world hunger, the resultant "fake food" has brought about more challenges and problems. Furthermore, compromising quality for the sake of quantity has

---

[37] Wahls, 2020.

led to increasing health problems such as cancer, autoimmunity, obesity and diabetes.

Fake foods are highly addictive. Children, and adults too, can't get enough of them. But these foods lack sufficient nutrients, plus nutrients are lost by the body in its effort to digest them. If you have ever wondered why you lack the energy to get out of bed or carry on your daily activities without sipping on coffee throughout the day, this is probably related to what you are eating. Existing on flour and sugar will leave you perpetually hungry and exhausted. In addition, it will kill your appetite for nutritious foods such as vegetables. For as long as you are addicted to fake foods, you are never likely to give vegetables a chance.

I have to admit that the more I learned about nutrition and food production, the more frustrating shopping became. Grocery stores have now become my gym for strengthening my willpower. In fact, if my will and perseverance could be turned into muscles, I would be Ms. Olympia!

There are so many foods to choose from, so many options on the shelves, and most of them taste amazingly delicious. I allow myself none of them. They are not real food. They are all fake food, containing many calories, but hardly any of the nutrients required by the body. If some product does contain a handful of added nutrients, that minuscule amount is not even worth the output of energy it takes to digest it. Packaged in the most appealing ways, this fake food is often falsely advertised. Many times I have picked up a new product because of a label that says "keto" or "no added sugar," only to read in the list of ingredients that an unhealthy sugar substitute has been added instead. So many products fall into this category, which is quite disheartening.

However, I urge you to start paying close attention to every product you consume. Is it fake food, or is it real? Will it nourish your body, or will it deplete it? If it's something with an ingredient list, research each word you do not understand. Don't buy anything you haven't researched.

Also, be sure to read the entire list of ingredients. They are listed in descending order by weight. The heaviest are listed first, so the first three ingredients stated should give you an idea of the main makeup of the product. Read the entire list, since producers may use different types of sugar to divide the weight and manipulate the order of the listing. Don't just look at the nutrition facts label.

Notice, for example, that the nutrition facts may state zero sugars, but cane sugar may be listed under the ingredients. If the amount of sugar in a serving is less than 0.5 grams, FDA labeling requirements allow the nutrition facts to state that there are zero grams. Since the "serving size" is usually much less than an average person would consume at one sitting, paying attention to all the ingredients is essential.

If it seems like a lot of work—good, because the mental process and time required to examine lengthy lists of ingredients will deter you from the unhealthiest products out there!

Another way of saving time when shopping is bypassing 80 percent of what's on offer and going directly to natural foods, which have no ingredient list. I have found doing this that the store shrinks in size, and so do my frustrations. No time gets wasted on reading and looking up words I don't understand. Through this simple process of elimination, the whole experience becomes effortless.

Food Coma and Coffee Dependence

A food coma is the feeling of being very tired or sleepy after eating a large, heavy meal. It happens because when you eat a big meal, your body needs to send more blood to your stomach and intestines to help digest the food. With more blood going to your digestive system, there is less blood going to other parts of your body, like your brain. This lack of blood flow to the brain can make you feel drowsy and sluggish. Eating foods high in trans fats, also called hydrogenated or partially hydrogenated oils, and processed carbohydrates makes a food coma more likely. To avoid a food coma, eat

LISTENING TO THE BODY'S NEEDS

small, lighter meals instead of overeating. Staying hydrated and going for a short walk after eating, can also help fight off that tired feeling.

Most of us know how a food coma feels, but not many know how it feels to live without it. The same goes for coffee; most can only function with it, but not without it. To discover new ways of living, we have to give up the old ways. We must detox. Just as it is healthy to minimize our possessions, the same principles apply when adopting a new lifestyle. Change must be more than superficial; we must get to the heart of the matter. There is no easy way out. To create space for the new, we must rid ourselves of the old.

How often we limit ourselves by how we think and what we do! We shovel down whatever comes our way to appease our hunger, since we don't have time to do otherwise. Then, to counteract the sleepiness caused by the food we just gorged on, we drink coffee – there is still so much work ahead of us – little realizing that our efforts to be more efficient are producing the opposite effect.

This can be compared to obtaining energy on credit: a credit card in the form of coffee. We drink coffee as we would swipe a credit card, borrowing energy when we don't have enough, only to have to pay it back in the future. The more coffee we drink, the more energy debt we accumulate. We feel energy-impoverished, exhausted.

How can we stop living on coffee credit?

Simple: Stop drinking the stuff! Stop buying on credit. Stop borrowing energy on credit. It is now time to repay the debt, which means giving back the borrowed energy. How? By sleeping and resting!

That's right. We allow ourselves the unthinkable: sleep and rest.

How? I can't tell you. You figure it out. Prioritize and put it on top of your list. When you do, your life and efficiency will be transformed and upgraded to another level.

Now, there are times when taking out a coffee loan is necessary, perhaps when we're at work or at school, but we must make sure we pay it back as soon as possible. Don't keep taking out more loans until the body declares bankruptcy. Body bankruptcy is different from the financial kind, in that it may be irreversible. What is lost may be lost forever. The resulting disease may still be managed effectively, but it may never completely disappear.

The Restart Detox

Five basic tastes have been identified: sweet, sour, salty, bitter, and umami. Each of them is responsible for assuring different survival functions. You may be unfamiliar with the term *umami*. It refers to a savory, meaty taste found in certain foods, such as tomatoes, mushrooms, soy sauce, Parmesan cheese and some meats. Umami adds depth and deliciousness to many dishes by bringing a richer, more complex flavor.

Sweet taste is responsible for ensuring the adequate intake of carbohydrates, which provide quick energy, whereas a bitter taste originally warned us against poisonous substances. Since we rarely consume bitter foods anymore, we have lost the ability to know what is toxic and what isn't. What a pity that harmful substances like high fructose corn syrup, added to nearly everything, are sweet and not bitter. If they were, we would instantly know that they are making us sick.

We are conditioned to prefer sweet tastes, but the body runs more efficiently when different flavors are introduced, and when our diets are diversified and well-balanced. The problem is, because we consume so much sugar and sweet-tasting foods, we have no way of knowing anything different, since it is outside our experience.

Just suppose you want to see how marvelous you can feel – how sharp your mind can be. Suppose you wish to experience a surge in energy that you have never experienced before. In that case, the only sugars you should consume should be those occurring naturally in fruit and vegetables. (Yes, vegetables contain sugars: in Europe, during World War II, jam and marmalade were made with swedes rutabagas!) You must give up processed foods with added sugars, and move away from all foods artificially enhanced with harmful substances. In their place, start eating fruit and vegetables superfoods!

Detoxing is not easy. It takes willpower and determination, but the results are well worth the effort. It will keep you away from hospitals!

Should dieting and refraining from comfort foods not be your strong suit (as for most of us), I urge you to find a buddy. Dieting together splits the effort in half, providing the same excellent results to both of you. Beginning is the tough part. You can't have the foods you're used to eating. Many of us turn to comfort foods, such as those made with flour and sugar, in response to stress. We come to associate certain foods with emotional relief. Breaking this emotional pattern of over-consumption can be particularly difficult.

You will probably find that, for the first four or five days, your mind turns constantly to the foods you crave. After that, be assured that these cravings will lessen significantly. You will start feeling the benefits of "eating clean." Give yourself much-deserved credit, for the worst and most challenging part is over.

But, before you start, let's get some of the misinformation sorted out.

The Fat-Free Diet Disaster

Throughout this book, I try to stress the importance of having an open mind. Scientific research is constantly evolving and at times new science debunks previously held beliefs. Such is the case with fat-free diets.

The trend of eating fat-free started in the mid-20th century after increased rates of heart disease were noticed in the US. People, including influential officials, wanted to know why, so they turned to science. The pressure was on to come up with answers. Much of the credit for providing them was given to Ancel Benjamin Keys, an American physiologist who conducted studies to learn the influence of diet on health. His Seven Country Study linked consumption of fat to higher levels of heart disease. This gave rise to new governmental dietary guidelines that suggested reducing fat intake as a means of combating this problem.

The food industry responded to these guidelines by producing low-fat and fat-free products. They substituted fat with sugar and refined carbohydrates from corn, soy and wheat. These crops were heavily subsidized. This was the start of a trend that has extended over many years and throughout many countries. The effects of Key's study continued well beyond his research.

In the intervening years we have learned that in spite of lowering the amount of fat in our diet, heart disease is still prevalent; in fact, it has increased. Along with even higher rates of heart disease, we now suffer from increased rates of other diseases like obesity, type 2 diabetes, metabolic syndrome, non-alcoholic fatty liver disease (NAFLD) and hypertension.

The intention was good – noble even – but the outcome did not work out as expected. Since Dr Key's conclusion has proved invalid, his study has now been scrutinized. This has revealed manipulation of the data. Results from a country that did not support his conclusion were simply disqualified.

It is very hard to reverse the impact of misinformation. Even after the release of recent scientific facts about healthy fats, I still hear people justify eating unhealthy snacks by saying that they are fat-free.

It Isn't the Fat and It's Not the Cholesterol

Cholesterol is an essential molecule without which there would be no life.[38]

---

[38] *The Great Cholesterol Myth Book.* Bowden & Sinatra, 2015.

Cholesterol is essential for many vital functions in the body. It is the precursor to sex hormones like estrogen, testosterone, and DHEA, as well as adrenal hormones, which regulate stress, water balance, and inflammation. When the skin is exposed to sunlight, cholesterol is converted to Vitamin D, which supports bone and immune health. Cholesterol, although demonized, actually aids the digestion of fats and fat-soluble vitamins (A, D, E, and K). It is critical for brain function. Furthermore, it insulates nerve fibers and facilitates the proper transmission of nerve impulses.

While cholesterol has been heavily emphasized as a risk factor for heart disease, emerging research suggests that by regulating inflammation and supporting overall physiological balance, cholesterol actually protects against heart disease and certain types of cancer. It is the balance of cholesterol levels that's essential, as both high and low cholesterol can pose health risks. Notably, approximately 50% of individuals who develop heart disease have cholesterol levels that fall within the normal range. Conversely, around 50% of people with elevated cholesterol levels show no signs of heart disease. Additionally, studies indicate that merely lowering cholesterol levels provides extremely limited benefits in terms of reducing heart disease risk or improving cardiac health.[39] These findings highlight that heart disease likely results from a complex interplay of various factors beyond just cholesterol levels alone.

In science, as we learn more, things become less simple than originally thought. Just as it is now known that not all fats are equally harmful, we also now know that some types of cholesterol are more harmful than others. In terms of fats, the harmful ones are trans fats (also called hydrogenated or partially hydrogenated oils) as well as highly processed or so-called refined oils like vegetable, canola, corn, and safflower oils. Other types of fat, however, are essential to life and lower inflammation. As for cholesterol, researchers have discovered that it is the LDL subtype B, which corresponds with high triglycerides, that increases the likelihood of heart disease. Some studies suggest that a low-fat, high-carbohydrate

---

39 Bowden & Sinatra, 2015.

diet – long promoted as heart-healthy – may actually increase harmful cholesterol levels. These studies indicate that fat, particularly saturated fat, helps reduce the number of small, dense LDL particles.

Inflammation Acute vs Chronic

Acute inflammation or an inflammatory response can occur after a sudden trauma. It is the body's attempt to repair the damage. The area concerned is often visible, since it gets red, swollen, and hot to the touch as a result of our immune system fighting off danger to the body. But if the injury is less obvious but persists for a long time, the inflammation may become chronic.

In the case of chronic inflammation, the cause may not be the result of an obvious visible injury. It could be provoked by certain foods that you've consumed all your life, or the cosmetics you have applied. Chronic inflammation may be going on in your body without you being aware of it, being a precursor to most diseases, such as the development of plaque buildup in the arteries (atherosclerosis). It inflicts harm on our vascular system, as well as vital organs like the brain, and other bodily tissues.[40]

As doctors Bowden & Sinatra succinctly put it in *The Great Cholesterol Myth Book*:

Acute inflammation hurts, chronic inflammation kills.

When inflammation is present in the body, a substance called C-reactive protein (CRP) is produced by the liver. The standard CRP test measures high levels of this protein in the blood, indicating the presence of significant inflammation. However, a high-sensitivity CRP (hs-CRP) test exists that is designed to detect even minor elevations of CRP in the bloodstream, which may not be apparent using the standard CRP test. Elevated hs-CRP

---

40   *Smart Fat Book*, Masley & Bowden, 2016.

levels are associated with an increased risk for heart attacks and strokes, even in individuals with normal cholesterol levels.

Understanding Fats

Over the years we have come to know much more about fats than was known back in the 1950s. Omega-6 fatty acids, found in junk food often made with vegetable oil, are pro-inflammatory whereas omega-3 fatty acids found in olives, olive oil, avocados, and most nuts are anti-inflammatory.

To effectively counteract inflammation, omega-3 and omega-6 fatty acids should be consumed in an ideal ratio of approximately 1:1. However, research shows that the predominant consumption of omega-6 fats is about 16 times greater than our consumption of omega-3s, resulting in a ratio of approximately 16:1. This imbalance means that we're providing 1,600 percent more "fuel" to the body's inflammatory processes than to its anti-inflammatory processes.

To simplify the understanding of fats, we can categorize them into three groups: good or smart fats (such as omega-3s), bad fats (such as certain saturated and trans fats), and neutral fats (such as monounsaturated fats).

Here is what Dr. Steven Masley and Dr. Bowden in their book *Smart Fat: Eat More Fat, Lose More Weight, Get Healthy Now* say about the bad (or dumb) kind, found in fast and packaged foods:

> Also called hydrogenated or partially hydrogenated oils, trans fats are biochemically similar to liquid plastic, essentially acting like embalming fluid in your tissue. Trans fats might lengthen a food's shelf life, but they will shorten your shelf life.

To avoid using unhealthy oils, which are high in omega-6 fats, and increase our use of omega-3 rich ones, we should limit ourselves to good quality olive oil for cold dishes and low-heat cooking. Coconut oil, or good-quality butter or ghee, should be used for high-heat cooking. I stress *good quality* because a lot of the olive oils in the stores are diluted and make misleading claims in their advertisements. Research before you buy.

Also, it is good to make sure that the butter and meat you use comes from grass-fed, grass-finished animal sources. Grass-finished means that the animal was not fattened up with corn six months before killing, to increase its weight and profit. Be sure to buy meat organically raised, without antibiotics and added growth hormones.

Doctors Masley & Bowden also advise us to steer clear of so-called vegetable oils:

> *Vegetable oils don't come from vegetables, so the name is misleading. They are processed from grains such as corn or from other plants such as soybeans. To distinguish these fats from animal fats manufacturers have long referred to them as vegetable oil.... But the name is flat-out wrong. More accurately they are plant-based oils derived from grains and seeds.*

The process of extracting them involves using harsh chemicals like hexane, benzene, acetone, and methylene chloride.

The Whole30 Program

The Whole30 program has changed my health in ways I could not have imagined were possible. I had never tested my hs-CRP levels, but knew I had inflammation in my body. I was in constant pain from acid reflux, had contact dermatitis that would present itself with all sorts of skin rashes, and often felt ill. If I encountered someone suffering from an infectious disease, I knew I would be getting it next. Perplexed by all these symptoms, I would consult my friend who is also a nurse and who would advise me to do the Whole30 clean-out program. She suspected I was reacting to certain foods that were making me sick.

I didn't know anything about the Whole30 program back then, but after I looked it up online, I was not inclined to find out more. No bread, no pasta, not even rice! No cheese, no milk, and no sugar! No chocolate! Forget it! I was not about to give up all the things I enjoyed eating. I dismissed her recommendation until my stomach pain and skin issues had become so unbearable that I was willing to try whatever possible to stop it.

The results were incredible! Not only did the heartburn and skin issues subside, but for the first time in my adult life I felt full of energy. I required less sleep to feel rested and did not need my usual naps on my days off. My skin looked healthy and radiant. My premenstrual cramping pains lessened. I lost 10 pounds. I felt so great that I continued to eat the Whole30 way many weeks past the 30 days that is recommended.

Reintroducing foods slowly has helped me identify those that had been making me sick throughout my life; foods that others may consider healthy. It's been 10 years now since I changed my eating habits after the Whole30 program. I eat very differently and don't ever get acid reflux. This doesn't mean that I don't ever eat bread, pasta, rice, milk, cheese or sweets; furthermore, I eat dark chocolate almost every day! What it means is that I have learned the language of my body. I now know how to recognize and understand the subtle messages it is communicating. I know how to balance foods I allow myself to eat on occasion with healthy fats, fruits, and vegetables that counteract the damage.

The Keto Diet

If you want to further your experience and challenge yourself even more, try the *Keto* diet. A ketogenic (keto) diet is a low-carbohydrate, high-fat diet designed to encourage the body to enter a state of ketosis. Ketosis occurs when there is a significant reduction in carbohydrate intake (sugars and starches), or when fasting. It means that instead of carbohydrates, the body primarily uses fat for energy, breaking down stored fat into molecules called ketones. The brain and other tissues use these ketones for energy. To reach and maintain ketosis, it's important not to over-consume protein, as excess protein can be converted into glucose, potentially interfering with ketosis.

The benefits of eating this way can include weight loss, improved blood sugar control and increased energy levels. It has been used as a therapeutic diet for conditions like epilepsy, and has gained popularity for weight loss and metabolic health.

Keto-Mojo is a blood ketone and glucose monitoring system. It is very useful for people to ensure that they stay in ketosis. The Keto-Mojo system typically includes a meter, lancets, and test strips for both blood ketone and glucose measurements. Users can take a small blood sample from a finger prick, then measure their ketone and glucose levels to track their state of ketosis and monitor their blood sugar. With this information they can adjust their diet and lifestyle to maintain ketosis and manage their blood sugar levels effectively. For people with type II diabetes, this diet is especially beneficial. It helps insulin-dependent patients to get off insulin and maintain their blood glucose levels within normal ranges.

The Wahls Paleo Plus Protocol

There is much misconception about the keto diet and how to follow it correctly. The Wahls Paleo Plus protocol is a refined keto diet; an anti-inflammatory diet like Whole30, combined with keto. Thanks to Dr. Wahls, we now know how to mix healthy essential fats with vegetables to keep ourselves in ketosis.

I once coached a patient with diabetes mellitus type II who initially injected insulin three times a day, taking 208 units daily, yet still often suffered severe consequences from fluctuating critical values. Despite taking that much insulin, her blood glucose readings would peak in the 300s, and would drop into the 60s. Within one month of starting the Wahls Paleo

Plus protocol, she lowered her insulin requirements to 20-40 units on most days, and maintained blood sugar levels within the normal range. After a few months of implementing this diet, she now only needs insulin on some days; most of the time, she can maintain her blood glucose levels within normal ranges without any insulin whatsoever.

Besides needing far less insulin, she has come off other prescription medications, such as gabapentin, prescribed for nerve pain. Her peripheral neuropathy has improved significantly. Other benefits from this diet include her losing 50 pounds, sleeping better, having less anxiety, improved skin complexion, and having more energy throughout the day.

For those who have autoimmune issues, or food sensitivities which prevent them from consuming eggs or dairy, achieving and staying in ketosis is still possible. Using the Wahls Paleo Plus Protocol, they can correctly mix these healthy, essential fats and vegetables without needing eggs or dairy products and still keep themselves in ketosis.

Lectins

Gluten sensitivity is often talked about as the cause of inflammation in the body, but not so many people are aware of lectins. Lectins, like gluten, are a diverse group of proteins known to cause inflammation. Although they don't work in the same way, both gluten and lectins can cause a kind of chemical warfare in your body, depending on your sensitivity and your overall health. This results in inflammatory reactions which cause significant damage to your gut. The renowned cardiologist and heart surgeon, Dr. Steven Gundry explains in his book "The Plant Paradox: The Hidden Dangers in Healthy Foods That Cause Disease and Weight Gain" how these proteins are designed by nature to protect plants against pests, pathogens and predators, including humans.

It is important to know that lectins can be reduced or deactivated through proper food preparation. Soaking nuts, seeds, beans, and legumes helps to reduce them. Pressure-cooking beans and legumes is an especially effective way of reducing lectins, as are fermenting and sprouting them.

The Mediterranean Diet

Our diets are closely related to the region or climate we live in or where we were born. Until recently, before industrialization, whatever Mother Nature provided in a given region became the main source of feeding ourselves. The Mediterranean diet is particularly healthy because it evolved from the sunny Mediterranean regions such as North Africa, the Near East, Greece, Italy, and Spain. These warm and sunny climates provide an abundance of fresh, ripe fruits and vegetables all year round. In this diet there is very little need for processed foods, so it is a great way to eat.

Seafood, such as fresh fish is a staple of the Mediterranean diet. Fish is a great source of anti-inflammatory omega-3. The problem is that harvesting and consuming fresh fish, from traditional sources outside of the Mediterranean has become much more difficult. Industrialized fishing has severely damaged marine ecosystems and biodiversity. Bottom trawling, for example, involves dragging a heavy net along the seafloor, causing significant damage to the seabed, destroying coral reefs and seagrass, which are crucial habitats for new and emerging sea life.

Farm fishing was going to be a more sustainable way of producing fish that would counteract the damage of industrialized fishing, but as it turns out, the effects are not any better. Heavy chemicals, antibiotics and processed feeds, used to sustain large numbers of fish in restricted areas, are highly detrimental to their health. This poses major risks to those who choose to consume farmed fish. In addition, these fish farms are often located inside a larger body of water such as seas, lakes and rivers, where the fish are enclosed by nets. As the water is not separate, spraying chemicals affects not only the fish that are being farmed, but the entire ecosystem. There have been numerous instances where the nets break and the genetically modified farmed fish get loose, potentially endangering the existence of natural species by affecting their genetic makeup or spreading disease. So if you choose to consume fish, be mindful of the source.

LISTENING TO THE BODY'S NEEDS

Most importantly the foundation of the Mediterranean diet is abundant amounts of high-quality olive oil – or as Homer, the legendary Greek poet, famously described it: "liquid gold." This liquid gold continues to live up to its ancient name. Science has been proving its value throughout many areas of health, such as:

- Lowering LDL (low-density lipoprotein) cholesterol
- Improving blood flow
- Reducing blood pressure
- Lowering the risks of cardiovascular events
- Preventing neurodegeneration such as Alzheimer's
- Boosting memory and learning
- Inhibiting cancer cell growth and reducing DNA damage caused by oxidative stress
- Promoting healthy gut microbiome by fostering beneficial bacteria
- Reducing gut inflammation
- Reducing the risk of type 2 diabetes
- Reducing signs of aging
- Supporting skin hydration and elasticity
- Helping maintain bone density
- Reducing risk of osteoporosis
- Olive oil contains oleocanthal, a compound with effects similar to ibuprofen, which helps reduce chronic inflammation.
- It contains polyphenols which suppress inflammatory markers, reducing the risk of diseases like arthritis and metabolic syndrome.
- Despite being calorie-dense it is associated with better weight control.

For maximum benefit, use extra virgin olive oil. Look for high polyphenol content on the label. Look for cold-pressed and stored in a dark glass bottle. If possible, choose unfiltered olive oil with lots of sediment on the bottom. The freshest is always best, so pay attention to the harvest dates stated on the label and choose those from within the last 12-18 months for best quality.

I once spoke to a friend of mine who grew up in a region of Italy – the Barbagia region of Sardinia – which is considered to be a Blue Zone. Blue Zones are regions where the rate of nonagenarians and centenarians is above the global average. These areas were identified by researcher Dan Buettner and his team in their studies of longevity around the world. My friend would reminisce about the fresh-cooked meals, always drenched in olive oil, which was filling and readily available.

The Magic of Cooking

When I look back at my early childhood, I remember much of our pretend play revolved around cooking. We mimicked in play what we observed in real life – the things that seemed important to everyone around us. Harvesting quality ingredients for our pretend dishes was a top priority. Since it was known that stinging nettle—a common weed that grows all over Poland—was good for us, we often used it to make our healthy pretend soups.

But harvesting stinging nettle is no easy task since, as the name implies, the plant is covered with little hairs that sting. Nettle stings produce painful bumps on the skin which can last from a few minutes to a few days, depending on the variety. My cousin and I would find creative ways to pick nettles without getting stung. The challenge of doing this made it even more fun. Then, we would use stones to grind them down, extracting the juices. After all that hard work, we added water, a few pinches of sand, plus whatever else we could find and voilà—dinner was served!

As I got older and was allowed to use real ingredients that I could put in my mouth and taste, my passion for cooking healthy dishes grew. Because I would always find a healthy substitute for less healthy ingredients, I was incapable of following the recipe book. My creations had no boundaries: from the most disgusting meat pancakes which I only made once – but which my sons still remember to this day – to the spinach brownies that left them puzzled. So many failures – but just as many successes!

LISTENING TO THE BODY'S NEEDS

Through years of cooking healthily, I have learned not to compromise taste in my quest for beneficial nutrients. When shopping for vegetables, I let myself be inspired by ethnic dishes from all over the world. I am particularly interested in those vegetables which are unfamiliar to me. Those with intriguing color and texture, from climates I've never experienced, are likely candidates to be the highlight of my evening dish. I use the internet to look up their names and learn everything I need to know to create my culinary masterpiece.

Cooking still feels like child's play to me. When shopping, I don't take a list but allow my intuition and curiosity to guide me. In this way, and with the help of the internet, a quick visit to the grocery store is transformed into an educational field trip. Fruits and vegetables from all parts of the world – what a variety! I marvel at all these nutrients, vitamins, and minerals in their purest form, without synthetic additives, grown in the soil of our Mother Earth. Pure medicine, all within our reach at the local market!

If only we could appreciate it more. Instead of sand, I can now use real spices like saffron, vanilla, cinnamon, cardamom, turmeric, paprika, cumin, cloves, allspice, anise, asafetida and coriander, among many others. To me, these spices are like colors to an artist. The difference is, I can see and eat the product of my creation.

The transformation that takes place while cooking food is multifaceted. Cooking is magical because how a chef feels at the time goes into what they cook. I believe it is not just the spices the chef puts in, but their attitude when they cook, which makes the flavor. Indeed, there are many styles of cooking. There is angry cooking, stressed cooking, slothful cooking, joyful cooking, exciting cooking, creative cooking, and passionate cooking. Each of these has its own style, but guess which has the best flavor? If you were to eat a meal consisting of any of the above, which one would you like to try? I'll take joy, excitement, creativity, and passion over anger, stress, and slothfulness any day!

You might think I'm crazy, but I've been cooking most of my life and have tested this theory repeatedly on my children. The kind of meal I produce depends on how I feel. It could be the same dish, which either everyone enjoyed or no one was feeling hungry. Its success or failure would be a reflection of my attitude.

Learning how to cook healthily not only keeps us in good physical shape but can also be an excellent form of therapy. Cutting, chopping, and stirring focus the attention and put us naturally into a state of mindfulness. As you gain confidence as a cook, you will see how the frustrations of the day magically melt away. Just as the simple ingredients of your dish are transformed, so are your feelings.

Engrossed in the act of cooking, let all your senses be stimulated. Be fully present while you cook, grateful for every ingredient you use. Pay close attention to details like temperature, texture, shape, color and smell, even with dishes you've made thousands of times, and you'll find that it will be a masterpiece on each occasion. Remind yourself before each meal that food is a gift of life. Transformed into energy, it sustains you and provides all your body requires.

Cooking is good for our mental health. With its sights, sounds, and smells, not only can it transform how we feel, but also it pervades the entire space around us. There is something wonderful about walking into a building where cooking is taking place. The whole atmosphere is inviting, the smells and warmth enticing. All our senses are awakened.

Although cooking can be time-consuming, it is never a waste of time. It is a lifelong investment in which the return is collected immediately by satisfying our hunger, and which becomes more valuable later in the form of resilience, agility, and the vibrancy we feel despite increasing birthdays.

The long-term benefits of cooking extend all through life. It is fundamental to good health. By cooking, I don't necessarily mean using heat, but mixing and combining fresh ingredients. This is the best way to detox. Make it yourself and you make it your own. This way, you can be certain about the quality of the food. The things you make most often are particularly significant since you consume them the most. Therefore, make your own vegetable dip or salad dressing, paleo or keto bread, bagels or buns, and almond flour, milk, or yogurt.

What To Eat

Your success in nutritional transformation lies not only in the things you eliminate from your diet but mostly in the new nutrient-dense things you learn to eat instead. Part of the detox process I recommend is going dairy-free for at least thirty days to observe changes within your digestive system and the way you feel. This is how I found out that I do not tolerate dairy products well and feel much better without them.

My favorite cheese alternatives are nutritional yeast and brewer's yeast, both derived from *Saccharomyces cerevisiae*. They are rich in B vitamins and minerals and can help reduce symptoms of Candida overgrowth.

DAIRY-FREE CHEESE SAUCE RECIPE

Servings:

4–6 people, 2–4 tablespoons per person

Ingredients:

- 1 cup cashews (soaked 2+ hours)
- ½ red bell pepper
- 4 tablespoons nutritional yeast
- 2 tablespoons hulled hemp seeds
- 2 ½ tablespoons lemon juice
- 1 ½ teaspoon Himalayan pink salt
- 1-2 cloves of garlic
- ¼ ½ medium size onion

Instructions:

1. Mix all ingredients together in a high-power blender.
2. May be used immediately added to soups, making them taste cheesy and creamy without the use of flour or dairy.
3. Cool in the refrigerator for 2-3 hours before serving as vegetable dip.

HOMEMADE ALMOND MILK RECIPE

Almond milk has become my favorite substitute for regular milk. I make my own to avoid the high content of preservatives in the store-bought kind. The perk of making almond milk yourself is the left-over almond pulp. This makes a great almond flour that can later be used for baking keto bread or buns.

Servings:

3–4 cups

Ingredients:

1 cup raw almonds

3-4 cups water

Instructions:

1. Soak the almonds: Place the almonds in a bowl and cover them with 2-3 cups of water. Let them soak overnight, or for at least 8 hours, to soften them.
2. Drain and rinse: After soaking, drain and rinse the almonds under cold water. You may want to peel the skins off.
3. Blend: Add the soaked almonds to a blender with 3-4 cups of fresh water. Blend on high until the almonds are completely pulverized and the mixture looks creamy (about 1-2 minutes).
4. Strain: Pour the almond mixture through a nut milk bag, cheesecloth or a fine-mesh strainer into a large bowl or pitcher. Squeeze or press to extract as much liquid as possible. This liquid is your almond milk.
5. Store the almond milk in an airtight container in the refrigerator for up to 4-5 days.

MAKING ALMOND FLOUR FROM ALMOND PULP

Instructions:

1. Dry the almond pulp: Spread the leftover almond pulp in a thin layer on a baking sheet. You can also use a dehydrator if you have one.

Oven method: Preheat your oven to the lowest setting (around 150-170°F or 65-75°C). Place the baking sheet in the oven and let the pulp dry for 2-4 hours, stirring occasionally, until it is completely dry and crumbly.

Dehydrator method: Set the dehydrator to 115°F (46°C) and let it run for 6-12 hours or until the pulp is completely dry.

2. Grind the pulp: Once the pulp is fully dried, break it into smaller pieces. Grind it into fine flour, using a blender, food processor or coffee grinder.

It is not easy to give up gluten and everything that contains it, especially when it comes to breads and buns. There are a lot of gluten-free breads on the market today, but they often contain substitute flours such as rice, corn, tapioca and potato, which will raise your blood glucose quickly and are not recommended during a detox program. It's best to avoid buying the substitutes and start baking your own bread and buns. Keto breads are an excellent choice since they are made with nut flours that contain anti-inflammatory essential fats and won't spike your blood sugar. As well as using nutritional yeast for its cheesy taste, another of my great discoveries since changing my eating habits has been psyllium husk, which imparts gluten-like elasticity to bread dough. It is a natural fiber that absorbs water and forms a gel-like substance, improving the dough's elasticity and texture.

KETO NUT BREAD RECIPE

Servings:

10–12

Ingredients:

- 2 cups almond flour
- 1/4 cup coconut flour
- 1/2 cup mixed nuts (chopped)
- 1/4 cup flaxseed meal (grind just before use, to avoid the loss of nutrients through oxidation)
- 1/4 cup psyllium husk powder
- 1 teaspoon baking soda
- 1/2 teaspoon salt
- 4 large eggs
- 1/2 cup melted coconut oil or ghee
- 1/2 cup unsweetened almond milk
- 1.5 tablespoon apple cider vinegar

Instructions:

1. Preheat your oven to 350°F (175°C). Grease a loaf pan or line it with parchment paper.
2. In a large bowl, combine the almond flour, coconut flour, chopped nuts, flaxseed meal, psyllium husk powder, baking soda, and salt.
3. Mix well to ensure even distribution.
4. In a separate bowl whisk together the eggs, melted coconut oil or ghee, almond milk and apple cider vinegar, until fully combined.
5. Pour the wet ingredients into the dry ingredients.

6. Stir until you get a thick batter.
7. Let the batter sit for a few minutes, to allow the psyllium husk and flaxseed to absorb moisture.
8. Spoon the batter into a prepared loaf pan, smoothing the top with a spatula.
9. Bake in the preheated oven for about 45-55 minutes, or until a toothpick inserted into the center comes out clean. If the top of the bread is browning too quickly, cover it with aluminum foil during the last 10-15 minutes of baking
10. Let the bread cool in the pan for about 10 minutes, then transfer it to a wire rack to cool completely.

KETO BUNS RECIPE

Servings:

6-8 buns

Ingredients:

- 2 cups almond flour
- 1/4 cup coconut flour
- 1/4 cup psyllium husk powder
- 1 teaspoon baking soda
- 1/2 teaspoon salt
- 2 large eggs
- 1/4 cup melted coconut oil or ghee
- 1/2 cup warm water
- 1&1/2 tablespoons apple cider vinegar
- 1 tablespoon sesame seeds (optional, for topping)

Instructions:

1. Preheat your oven to 350°F (175°C). Line a baking sheet with parchment paper or lightly grease it.
2. In a large bowl combine the almond flour, coconut flour, psyllium husk powder, baking soda and salt. Mix well to ensure even distribution.
3. In a separate bowl whisk together the eggs, melted ghee (or coconut oil), warm water, and apple cider vinegar until fully combined.
4. Combine ingredients: Pour the wet ingredients into the dry ingredients. Stir until you get a thick dough. Let the dough sit for a few minutes to allow the psyllium husk and other ingredients to absorb moisture.

5. Shape the buns: Divide the dough into 6-8 equal portions, depending on the size of the buns you want. Roll each portion into a ball and flatten it slightly to form bun shapes. Place them on the prepared baking sheet.
6. Add toppings (optional): If desired, sprinkle the tops of the buns with sesame seeds for extra flavor and texture.
7. Bake in a preheated oven for 20-25 minutes or until the buns are golden brown and a toothpick inserted into the center comes out clean.
8. Cool: Allow the buns to cool on the baking sheet for 10 minutes, then transfer them to a wire rack to cool completely.
9. Serve: Slice and enjoy your keto buns! Store any leftovers in an airtight container at room temperature for up to 2 days, or in the refrigerator for up to a week. They also freeze well for up to 3 months.

If your sweet tooth is as large as mine, you will need to find healthy substitutes to satisfy your cravings for sweets, especially in the early stages of your detox. As you make progress, you will observe your sweet tooth significantly shrinking in size.

In baking, bananas make a great sugar substitute. Unripe bananas, although less sweet than the ripe ones, are especially healthy for their high amount of resistant starch, and act as dietary fiber.

In addition, using keto dark chocolate powder is a great way to curb your cravings for sweets. Keto chocolate has a higher cocoa butter content than regular chocolate, so it is a great source of healthy fats in addition to its high content of flavonoids. Use it in your brownies and even to make your own chocolate, after you finish your detox. The bitterness of any 70 percent (or higher) chocolate should deter you from overindulging. As you develop a new appreciation for this acquired taste, you will find that even a small amount can satisfy the largest cravings.

HEALTHY BROWNIE RECIPE

Servings:

8-12 squares

Ingredients:

- 3 bananas
- 1 cup nut butter
- ½ cup unsweetened keto cacao powder

Optional:

- ½ cup pine nuts
- 3 Medjool dates (to increase sweetness)
- ¼ cinnamon or other spices

Instructions:

1. Preheat your oven to 350°F (175°C).
2. Grease an 8-inch square baking dish or line it with parchment paper.
3. In a large bowl, mash the bananas with a fork until smooth.
4. Add the nut butter, cocoa powder, and the rest of the optional ingredients. Mix until fully combined.
5. Spoon the batter into the prepared baking dish, smoothing the top with a spatula.
6. Bake in the preheated oven for about 20-25 minutes, or until set.
7. Let it cool for about 15 minutes before serving.

The Takeaways:

- Look around your kitchen and see what you can substitute for a healthier choice.
- Start preparing for your 30-day whole foods challenge.
- Set up a perfect date to start and follow through on it.
- See if any of your friends would like to join in on the idea!

Chapter 7

Holistic Eating

Food can be the most powerful form of medicine or the slowest form of poison.

Ann Wigmore

Think of yourself as an investor, your body as a mutual fund, your lifestyle as your fund manager and the foods you eat as currency. Depending on your lifestyle, the "assets" you choose to eat or "invest in" are incorporated into your body and become your mutual fund. How you manage your "portfolio" and the quality of foods or "securities" you choose, determines the returns you're able to generate. These returns are passed back to you in the form of energy that in turn gets collected as successful aging. Sounds like a wonderful 401K plan to me!

Rather than concentrating on our financial health, let's not overlook the one invaluable asset that makes it all possible – our body.

What are Nourishing Foods?

From now on, **nourished** is how you want to be. No snacking on trashy foods, even if it means being hungry for a while. Before you put anything in your mouth, ask yourself if it is nourishing or trash. When in doubt, leave it.

If you want to detox, but so far your attitude is for food to merely taste good and nothing else, you will have no clue what is right to eat. Up to now, poor quality food is all you've ever known. You probably think I'm exaggerating, but a salad dressed with a long list of ingredients including high fructose corn syrup is still harmful to our body. Broccoli cooked in vegetable oil, smeared all over with processed cheese, should never be allowed to make it to the healthy foods section.

HOLISTIC EATING

The problem is, we fail to recognize that 'healthy' is often destroyed by 'unhealthy.' Most likely, you have no idea how bad your food makes you feel. The doctor might diagnose your diseases without ever tying any of them back to the root cause – the unhealthy foods you're eating.

To ensure your success at this life-changing detox, and to keep you away from the hospital, it is not enough to know what not to eat; you must know what to eat in its place. If you are unprepared, with no replacement foods at hand, you will feel hunger cravings and grab anything familiar. Preparation is the key to success, especially since now you can't eat out! That's right no eating out, since no restaurant can be trusted to have solely YOUR health interests at heart. From now on, you must prepare your own meals and plan them ahead of time.

Eating raw foods is a great alternative. Primarily, raw foods haven't been damaged by cooking, so they remain enzyme-rich and nutrient-dense. If you are new to raw foods, or cringe at the idea, you might not be ready. Your digestive system might revolt since it has never been nourished this way before. At first, you may lack the digestive enzymes needed; progress slowly, trying a little at a time. Don't be discouraged when your body initially rejects raw food. It will take time for you to get used to the idea of food as medicine. After a while, the unthinkable will happen. You will be craving healthy foods, grabbing raw broccoli, cauliflower or peppers for a snack.

Navigate the healthcare system's challenges by prioritizing your well-being with organic vegetables, fruits, sprouts, soaked nuts and seeds, and green smoothies. Even if you find yourself in it – since not everything is preventable – you will have a short stay and a speedy recovery.

Incidentally, most nuts and seeds should be pre-soaked since their skins can be harmful or difficult to digest. To make them crispy again and to preserve their nutrition, dehydrate them either in a food dryer, or in an oven at 150 – 170 degrees Fahrenheit.

Making Healthy Affordable

Efforts to motivate my co-workers, friends and family to change their lifestyle and unhealthy eating habits often get shot down with: "*It's too expensive.*"

It's true: eating healthy can be very expensive, but there are ways to make it affordable. Growing your own food in the garden is best, but often not an option if you live in an inner city. Having said that, I've seen some incredible vegetables grown in pots on balconies and patios, and herbal gardens decorating inner-city kitchens. The next best thing is to buy local foods in season. These taste best and are often discounted before they can spoil and waste.

When I come across a great deal on seasonal produce, I usually buy in bulk and find ways to preserve it, just as my grandmother used to do. In the summertime, she was often left with a surplus of delicious produce from her garden and had to find different ways to keep it for the long winters to come.

Fruits like blueberries, black and red currants, cherries, pears and tomatoes can be placed in special preserving (Mason) jars, covered with water and heated in the oven for about twenty minutes to make a good seal. Make doubly sure you seal your jars correctly to prevent air getting in. This no-air environment is essential to keep the food fresh and stop bacteria and mold from growing. Fruits correctly preserved in these jars will last throughout the year and are a wonderful and healthy treat to open on winter days, or special holidays like Christmas. Vegetables like onions, beets, peppers and cauliflower are also great for preserving. The process is very similar to that of preserving fruits, but may require the addition of salt, herbs, spices and sometimes a bit of vinegar, for flavor and storing.

Other ways to preserve herbs, fruits, and vegetables are to freeze them, dry them or dehydrate them. One of my favorite ways of preserving garlic, turmeric and basil is to turn them into a pesto (paste) using a lot of good quality, unfiltered olive oil. I then keep them frozen in ice-cube containers – easy to add to my favorite soups and other dishes.

Preparation

Preparation is key to saving money. For example, frozen cauliflower rice may cost you five times more than buying the ingredients yourself and making your own version at home. When you buy a fresh cauliflower in season, chop it, and freeze it yourself. Produce that is conveniently rinsed, chopped and pre-cut comes at a premium price, just to save you some prep time. But if you plan your meals ahead, you can eat healthily and save money.

Pre-made soups and broths can be expensive, but they can also all be made at home and saved for later. All soups, even bone broth or chicken stock, if poured into a jar boiling hot, fresh off the stove and tightly closed with a stainless-steel lid, create a vacuum as they cool down. Preserved in this way, you can store them for another time. Fresh soups don't need to be frozen as this often impairs the taste. These soups are perfect for lunch at work.

If you find that, when you begin to eat healthy, it is costing you more than when you ate processed foods, it may be that you are not planning your meals efficiently and wasting a lot of food as a result.

Successful Detoxing

To be successful, you should detox fully for at least one month. If you decide to detox and spend a fortune on healthy organic foods, cook a delicious meal, then the next day eat out with friends, there is a high chance that much of what you have bought (and even prepared) will spoil and end up in the trash. Do that a couple of times a month and it becomes costly. You must be determined and consistent.

You may find that, because you have been in the habit of eating out, spending a significant amount at the grocery store comes as a shock. But trust me, the money you spend each day on individual meals and snacks adds up to a larger sum. Not to mention the diseases that result, and the associated hospital bills which may leave you broke anyway. You can't say eating healthy is too expensive if you don't take on the challenge, change your lifestyle and calculate your spending fairly.

Eating fake food might appear inexpensive in comparison, but it's a waste of money since it doesn't feed you properly; you're cheating your body out of nutrients. Yes, the feeling of hunger is taken away, but your digestive system works hard to break it down, and the energy delivered is poor quality. Children might be able keep going on fake food since they are young and resilient but, as we grow older, the body finds it more difficult to compensate for an inadequate diet.

Medicinal Soups and Bone Broth

Bone Broth

Bone broth is a clear, protein-rich liquid obtained by simmering meaty joints and bones in boiling water. Broth is distinguished from stock by its lengthy cooking time, but much like stock can be used as a base for soups, stews, and sauces. Its quality and health benefits are determined by the kind of meat used. For best results, select grass fed/grass finished bovine femur bones and joints, such as knuckles and feet, but you may add other bones from previously made chicken stock or meat dishes. Whenever you are cooking, save and freeze unused bones, using them later to make broth. Cooking slowly on a low heat with an acidic ingredient, such as a few tablespoons of apple cider vinegar, will enhance nutrient extraction.

The benefits of bone broth have been known for generations. Bone broth is rich in proteins, amino acids and minerals. Recent research is now revealing its potential to prevent and treat diseases caused by nutritional deficiencies, such as ulcerative colitis. The existing treatments for this disease involve prolonged use of anti-inflammatory drugs and immunosuppressants. These are costly, have limited efficacy and can cause adverse side effects. Further research will determine if consuming bone broth could be a natural, cost-effective alternative that yields results comparable to those achieved through gene and pharmacological therapies.[41] It's packed with vitamins and minerals that aid digestion and fight inflammation. Additionally, it has anti-aging effects due to collagen, improves joint health, sleep, brain function and supports weight loss.[42]

---

41   Mar-Soil et al., 2021.
42   Philpotts, 2023.

BONE BROTH RECIPE

Servings:

16-24 cups

Ingredients:

- 2-3 pounds of bones (beef, chicken, pork or a combination). Knuckles are particularly good.
- 4 chicken feet (optional but recommended)
- Any vegetables and spices used in the chicken stock recipe below, or any vegetables in your fridge that are getting a little bit limp.
- 2-3 tablespoons apple cider vinegar
- Salt and pepper to taste

Instructions:

1. Place the bones in a large pot. Pour in enough water to cover the ingredients by about 2 inches. Add the spices and apple cider vinegar (which helps extract minerals from the bones).
2. Bring the pot to a boil, then reduce the heat to a simmer. Skim off any foam that rises to the surface. Simmer for at least 12-24 hours. The longer it cooks, the more nutritious the broth will be.
3. Add vegetables about 4 hours before the end.
4. After cooking, remove the larger solids with a slotted spoon. Strain the broth through a fine-mesh sieve or cheesecloth into another pot or bowl.
5. Transfer into jars.
6. Store in the refrigerator for up to 14 days or freeze for longer storage (up to 3 months).
7. Enjoy the bone broth as a warm drink, use it as a base for soups, stews or sauces, or incorporate it into various recipes for added flavor and nutrients. Feel free to adjust the ingredients and cooking time based on your preferences and the type of bones you're using.

CHICKEN STOCK AND BEEF STOCK

Both chicken stock and beef stock are very nutritious, and provide an awesome base for many dishes.

Chicken Stock Recipe

I like to use a free-range chicken, reared naturally without the use of growth hormones, which is denser in muscle mass and will need more time to cook. Cooking time is, therefore, a good gauge of the quality of the meat.

Servings:

14-22 cups

Ingredients:

1 whole USDA organic chicken (or preferably from a local farm that you can visit and trust)

- 1 teaspoon black peppercorns
- 2-3 bay leaves
- 3-4 allspice berries
- 1 tablespoon salt (adjust to taste)
- 4-5 garlic cloves
- 1 large onion, cleaned, unpeeled
- 2-3 carrots, (including the carrot greens if available)
- 1 celery root, peeled
- 3-5 celery sticks
- 1 leek, cleaned, cut in half to fit your pot
- 2 parsley roots, peeled
- 1 bunch parsley leaves

- 1-2 sprigs lovage (or substitute with dill or cilantro if unavailable)
- 1/2 hot pepper (adjust to your spice preference)

Instructions:

1. Place the chicken in a large stockpot and add enough cold water to cover all the ingredients by about 2 inches. This is usually around 16-24 cups of water, depending on the size of your pot and the amount of ingredients.
2. Add spices: black peppercorns, bay leaves and allspice berries.
3. Heat and simmer: Bring the pot to the boil over a medium-high heat. Once it boils, reduce the heat to low and let it simmer gently. Skim off any foam or impurities that rise to the surface with a spoon.
4. Add the garlic cloves, onion, carrots, celery root, celery sticks, leek, parsley root, parsley leaves, lovage and 1/2 hot pepper to the pot.
5. Simmer for flavor: Let the stock simmer for at least 2-3 hours, preferably up to 4-6 hours for a richer flavor. The longer it simmers, the more flavors are extracted from the ingredients.
6. Add salt to taste.
7. Remove the pot from the heat. Using a ladle, pour the stock into preserving jars leaving about 1 inch of headspace at the top. Close the lid tight while wearing oven mitts.
8. Check the seals. After the jars have cooled, check the seal by pressing the center of each lid. If the lid does not flex up and down, the jar is sealed. If any jars did not seal properly, refrigerate them and use the stock within a few days.
9. Store in the refrigerator for up to 14 days or freeze for longer storage (up to 3 months).
10. Use and enjoy! Chicken stock as a base for soups, stews, sauces or any recipe calling for chicken broth or stock. Enjoy the rich, homemade Favor.

Notes:

Adjust the amount of salt and hot pepper according to your taste preferences. This chicken stock recipe is versatile and can be adapted to suit your taste and the ingredients you have on hand.

BEEF STOCK RECIPE

I make beef stock in a similar way to chicken stock.

Instructions:

1. First cook the meat with spices like black pepper, bay leaf, and allspice.
2. After the meat becomes tender, add the basic stock vegetables: whole onion (with its skin, included for the nutritional benefits); garlic; carrots; whole parsley, including the roots, stems and leaves; and whole celery, also including the root, stalks and leaves. If you have a leek, add one whole as well. Be sure to rinse it thoroughly between each of its layers where the dirt likes to reside.
3. Add a half or whole jalapeño pepper, depending on your preference that day.
4. At the very end of cooking, add salt to taste.

I use a huge stock pot, as any smaller pot will be insufficient to make enough stock for me to have some left for another day. Although, with the delicious smell pervading the entire house and surrounding neighborhood, it usually gets eaten faster than I can store it!

Soups in general are fabulous for their nutritional content and great for tight budgets. Cooking soups often allows me to use a lot of scraps of left-over vegetables that need to be used up – nothing gets thrown away. With preserved jars full of delicious and highly nutritious bone broth and chicken stock or vegetable stock as base, I can make any soup quickly, significantly cutting down on cooking time.

VEGAN AND VEGETARIAN SOUPS

Soups do not need to be based on animal products. Even though there are no true plant-based sources of collagen, plants can help boost the body's own collagen production by providing the necessary nutrients.

To make vegan and vegetarian soups, make vegetable broth in the same way as you would a bone broth or chicken stock, but substituting the meat with vegetables and all kinds of wonderful spices. You can use vegetables like onion, carrots, parsley, celery, garlic and leeks to make a base that can be transformed into other dishes. Don't be afraid to use vegetables with potent flavors such as mushrooms, lovage, dill, cilantro, basil and curry, keeping in mind they may dominate the flavor, will affect the taste of your other dishes. Spices are full of anti-inflammatory and antioxidants, so use them generously. Use any that you like, but some of my favorites are turmeric, coriander, cumin, ginger, fenugreek, cardamom, cloves, cinnamon, black pepper, mustard seeds and chili powder. Simmer down the liquid for a good while, so that all the delicious vegetable juices are released. Put in preserving jars, close the lid tightly, and store.

When you are ready to make your next vegetable soup, use your previously made vegetable broth or some good-quality olive, pickle, cabbage, or kimchi[43] brine. Each time you finish eating a jar of olives or pickles, do not toss that liquid out. Store it, to enrich the taste of your soups and other dishes.

Sauté your desired vegetables with spices in high-quality oil, like cold-pressed extra virgin coconut oil. Add water, and when all is fully cooked to your desired softness, as the last step, after turning off the heat, add the brine. Brine is salty, so do not add extra salt early on in your cooking. If necessary, add salt only after you've poured in the brine.

---

[43] Kimchi is a traditional Korean dish made from fermented vegetables, most commonly using cabbage or radishes, along with various seasonings like chili peppers, garlic, ginger, and salt. The ingredients are mixed together and left to ferment, resulting in a tangy, spicy, and flavorful dish.

Instead of brine, you could use miso,[44] a traditional Japanese seasoning. If you do this, discontinue cooking immediately to preserve the miso beneficial micro bacteria.

VEGAN/VEGETABLE BROTH (STOCK) RECIPE

Ingredients:

- Vegetables used in the chicken stock recipe (or whatever you have available)
- Spices used in the chicken stock recipe and any other that you like to use
- 1-2 cups mushrooms (optional for richer flavor)
- 1 sprig of fresh thyme or 1 teaspoon of dried thyme
- 1 sprig of fresh rosemary or 1 teaspoon of dried rosemary
- Salt to taste

Instructions:

1. Place all the vegetables and spices in a large pot and cover with water.
2. Bring the pot to a boil, then reduce the heat to simmer. Simmer uncovered for 2 hours.
3. Transfer to preserving jars using the same method as mentioned in the chicken stock recipe above.
4. Store the same way as you would a chicken stock or bone broth.

---

[44] Miso, is a traditional Japanese seasoning produced by fermenting soybeans with salt and koji (a type of fungus) along with other ingredients like rice, barley, or other grains. The mixture is aged for varying periods, ranging from a few months to several years, resulting in a thick paste with a complex, salty, and savory flavor.

VEGAN VEGETABLE SOUP RECIPE

Ingredients:

- 2-6 tablespoons olive oil
- Vegetables used in the chicken stock recipe (or whatever you have available)
- Spices used in the chicken stock recipe and any other that you like to use
- 6 potatoes
- Leftover olive brine (optional)
- Cheeseless cheese dip (optional)
- Salt to taste

Instructions:

1. Prepare the vegetables: Wash, peel, and roughly chop all the vegetables.
2. Sauté the vegetables: In a large pot, heat the olive oil over medium heat. Add spices, then add the vegetables. Sauté for about 10-15 minutes, until they start to soften and become fragrant.
3. Pour in the water to cover the vegetables.
4. Simmer: Bring the pot to a boil, then reduce the heat to a simmer. Simmer for at least 45 minutes to 1 hour. For a more intense flavor, simmer for up to 2 hours.
5. Remove the pot from the heat. Pour in the leftover olive brine, or a desired amount of the cheeseless cheese dip (recipe mentioned in the takeaways of chapter 6).
6. Taste the soup and add salt as needed.
7. Transfer to preserving jars, using the same method as mentioned in the chicken stock. You can keep the pot of soup in the refrigerator for up to 5 days.

You may like to try these other soups:

TOMATO SOUP RECIPE

For those sensitive to lectins, present in the skins and seeds of tomatoes, it is best to use tomato paste from which they have been sieved out. If you are using fresh tomatoes, allow them to boil for longer, using a higher heat to help break the lectins down.

Ingredients:

- 2 tablespoons olive oil or butter
- 1 large onion, finely chopped
- 2-3 cloves garlic, minced
- 1-2 cans tomato paste (6-12 ounces), or use 1.5-3 cups whole peeled tomatoes, crushed by hand
- 4-8 cups vegetable or chicken broth
- 1 teaspoon dried basil (or 1 tablespoon fresh basil, chopped)
- 1 teaspoon dried thyme (or 1 tablespoon fresh thyme leaves)
- Salt and pepper to taste
- 1/2 cup coconut cream (optional, for a creamy version)
- Fresh basil, dill, cilantro or parsley for garnish (optional)

Instructions:

1. Sauté the vegetables: In a large pot, heat the olive oil or butter over medium heat. Add the chopped onion and sauté for about 5-7 minutes until softened and translucent. Add the minced garlic and cook for another 1-2 minutes until fragrant.
2. Add the tomato paste or tomatoes: Stir in and cook for 2-3 minutes, allowing it to caramelize slightly and deepen in flavor.
3. Add broth: Pour in the premade broth and stir to combine.

4. Add the dried basil and the dried thyme.
5. Bring the mixture to a boil, then reduce the heat and let it simmer for about 20-30 minutes to allow the flavors to meld.
6. Blend the soup: Use an immersion blender to puree the soup until smooth. If you prefer a chunkier soup, blend only part of the soup or skip blending altogether.
7. Add cream (optional): If you want a creamy tomato soup, stir in the coconut cream.
8. Taste the soup and season with salt and pepper as needed.
9. Serve: Ladle the soup into bowls and garnish with fresh basil, dill, cilantro or parsley if desired.

This soup can be stored in the refrigerator for up to 5 days or frozen for up to 3 months.

Note: it can be served with rice or potatoes.

ONION AND LEEK SOUP RECIPE

Ingredients:

- 2 tablespoons olive oil or butter
- 4 large onions, thinly sliced
- 3 large leeks, white and light green parts only, thinly sliced
- 2-3 cloves garlic, minced
- 1 teaspoon dried thyme (or 1 tablespoon fresh thyme leaves)
- 1 bay leaf
- 6 cups vegetable or chicken broth
- Salt and pepper to taste
- 1/2 cup cheeseless cheese dip (recipe in chapter 6)
- Fresh parsley or chives for garnish (optional)

Instructions:

1. Prepare the leeks: Slice the leeks lengthwise and rinse them thoroughly under cold water to remove any dirt or sand. Pat them dry and slice thinly.
2. Sauté the onions and leeks: In a large pot, heat the olive oil or butter over medium heat. Add the sliced onions and leeks, stirring to coat them in the oil. Cook for about 10-15 minutes, stirring occasionally, until the onions and leeks are softened.
3. Add garlic and seasonings: Add the minced garlic and cook for another 1-2 minutes until fragrant. Stir in the dried thyme and bay leaf.
4. Add broth: Pour in the premade broth and stir to combine. Bring the mixture to a boil, then reduce the heat and let it simmer for about 20-30 minutes to allow the flavors to meld.
5. Add cheeseless cheese dip.

6. Season and blend (optional): Taste the soup, and season with salt and pepper as needed. If you prefer a smoother soup, you can use a blender to partially blend it, leaving some texture.
7. Serve: Ladle the soup into bowls and garnish with fresh parsley or chives if desired.

To make the soup more substantial, you can add cooked potatoes.

This soup can be stored in the refrigerator for up to 5 days or frozen for up to 3 months.

POLISH BORSCHT (BEET) SOUP

To make delicious beet soup or borscht (*barszcz*), as we call it in Poland, sauté whole beets, including the chopped up roots and leaves, with onion. Then add in the broth. Borscht needs a bit of lemon juice at the end for taste and to preserve its red color. You may also add coconut milk to make it even more flavorful and change its color to a beautiful pink.

Nutrient Dense Polish Barszcz (Borscht) Beet Soup Recipe

Ingredients:

- 2 tablespoons olive oil
- 1 pound (450g) grass-fed and grass-finished beef stew meat or beef shank, cut into chunks
- 1 large onion, finely chopped
- 2-3 cloves garlic, minced
- 4 medium beets with their leaves, peeled and cut into squares / grated (greens finely chopped)
- 3 large carrots, peeled and chopped/grated
- 3 medium potatoes, peeled and diced
- 6 cups premade broth
- 2 tablespoons apple cider vinegar or lemon juice
- 1 bay leaf
- Salt and pepper to taste
- Fresh dill or parsley, chopped (for garnish)
- Coconut cream (optional)

Instructions:

1. Brown the beef: In a pan, heat the olive oil over medium heat. Add the beef chunks and brown on all sides for about 5-7 minutes. Remove the beef, and set aside.
2. In the same pot, add the chopped onion and sauté for about 5 minutes, until it becomes translucent. Add the minced garlic and sauté for another minute until fragrant.
3. Add the beets and carrot: Add the grated beets and carrot to the pot. Cook for about 5-7 minutes, stirring occasionally, until they start to soften.
4. Combine ingredients: Return the browned beef to the pot. Pour in the premade beef broth. Add the diced potato and bay leaf. Bring the mixture to a boil, then reduce the heat to low and let it simmer for about 45 minutes to 1 hour until the beets are tender and the vegetables are cooked through.
5. Add beet leaves and seasonings: Stir in the finely chopped beet leaves. Add the apple cider vinegar or lemon juice. Season with salt and pepper to taste. Simmer for another 10-15 minutes to allow the flavors to meld.
6. Serve: Remove the bay leaf before serving. Ladle the borscht into bowls and garnish with fresh dill or parsley. Serve hot with a dollop of coconut cream.

Enjoy your hearty and nutritious Polish Borscht with beef and beet greens!

BEET KVASS

Beet kvass is a traditional, natural fermented drink rich in probiotics and vitamins. Kvass is often made from beets, rye bread, or other grains. It's a naturally carbonated drink rich in probiotics, typically consumed as a health tonic or for culinary purposes such as in borscht. Kvass is fermented using beneficial bacteria and yeasts, which turn sugars from natural ingredients like beets or bread into alcohol and organic acids, creating its characteristic sour, tangy flavor. It is usually drunk as a refreshing beverage, used as a base for soups, or in some dishes.

Kvass and brine are not the same, though they are related in the sense that both involve fermentation. Kvass is a beverage, while brine is a preservation medium.

Here's a simple recipe:

Ingredients:

- 1 kg (2.2 lbs) red beets (preferably organic)
- 1 liter (4 cups) boiled and cooled water
- 1-2 garlic cloves (optional)
- 1-2 bay leaves
- 3-4 allspice berries
- 1 teaspoon salt (preferably non-iodized, like rock salt or Himalayan) per 1 liter of water
- A piece of sourdough bread crust (optional, to speed up fermentation)

Instructions:

1. Prepare the Beets: Peel and slice the beets into thin slices or chunks. If using organic beets, you can wash them thoroughly and leave the skin on.

2. Layer Ingredients: Place the sliced beets in a large, clean, sterilized jar or ceramic fermentation crock. Add the garlic cloves (peeled), bay leaves, allspice, and optional sourdough bread (wrap it in cheesecloth for easy removal later).
3. Make the Brine: Dissolve the salt in the boiled, cooled water. Pour the salted water over the beets and other ingredients, ensuring everything is fully submerged. If the beets float, weigh them down with a clean plate or fermentation weight.
4. Fermentation Process: Cover the jar or crock with a clean cloth or loosely with a lid to allow air circulation but protect it from contaminants. Leave the jar in a warm, dark place (around 18–24°C/64–75°F) for about 5–7 days. The fermentation process will be faster in warmer conditions.
5. Daily Check: Check daily for any mold on the surface. If any appears, carefully remove it with a clean spoon. After a few days, the kvass will start to develop a deep red color and a tangy, earthy flavor.
6. Strain and Store: Once the kvass reaches the desired level of sourness (around 5–7 days), strain the liquid through a fine sieve. Pour the strained kvass into sterilized bottles or jars, seal tightly, and store in the refrigerator. It will keep for several weeks.

Tips:

If you don't use sourdough bread, the fermentation process may take a little longer but will still work perfectly. For extra flavor, you can add a piece of fresh ginger, horseradish, or a few cloves.

POLISH BORSCHT WITH BEET KVASS

Ingredients:

- Leftover beets from kvass (about 2-3 medium-sized beets)
- 1 medium onion, finely chopped
- 1 tablespoon olive oil (or butter)
- 1-2 wild mushrooms (optional, such as chanterelles or porcini, chopped)
- 1 bay leaf
- 1 teaspoon dried dill (or fresh dill if available)
- Salt and pepper to taste
- 2-3 cups of water or vegetable broth
- 2 cups beet kvass (adjust to taste)
- 1 tablespoon apple cider vinegar (optional, for extra tang)
- Fresh herbs for garnish (parsley or dill)

Instructions:

1. **Cook the Beets and Onion:** In a pot, heat the olive oil (or butter) over medium heat. Add the chopped onion and sauté until softened, about 5-7 minutes.
2. **Add Mushrooms and Spices:** If using, add the wild mushrooms and cook for an additional 3-5 minutes until they soften and release their flavor. Stir in the bay leaf and dried dill.
3. **Add the Leftover Beets:** Add the leftover beets from your kvass to the pot. Stir to combine with the onion and mushrooms.
4. **Add Liquid and Simmer:** Pour in 2-3 cups of water or vegetable broth, then bring to a simmer. Let it cook for about 10 minutes to allow the flavors to blend.

5. Let the soup cool slightly for a few minutes, then stir in the kvass just before serving or once the pot has been removed from the heat. This way, the kvass will retain its probiotics, and you'll get all the benefits of the fermentation. Adjust the amount of kvass based on your desired level of sourness.
6. Add salt and pepper to taste. If you'd like more acidity, add apple cider vinegar.
7. Serve: Ladle the borscht into bowls, and garnish with fresh herbs like parsley or dill. Serve with a dollop of sour cream.

Tips:

If you want a richer borscht, you can add more mushrooms or even a spoonful of sauerkraut for added tang. This recipe is flexible, so feel free to adjust the spices or liquid to suit your taste. Borscht is often better the next day, as the flavors have more time to develop.

The borscht and its key ingredient kvass made this way is full of probiotics, antioxidants, fiber, and vitamins that support gut health, detoxification, immune function, blood pressure regulation, and more. In addition, both kvass and borscht are delicious, making it a fun and easy way to improve your overall health!

The Trash Reward

One way to know if you are on the right path to holistic eating is by watching your trash. That's right! Your new lifestyle will significantly affect what you throw away. This should change from a large amount of inorganic plastic wrapping to a significantly smaller amount of compostable organic matter. If there is somewhere you can put a compost bin, you have the ability to compost and I urge you to do so. You will see that eating clean is also great for the environment, and notice that you barely produce any trash at all. The trash cans, previously full to the brim, getting filled up too quickly for the garbage company to keep up, won't need to be taken out so frequently.

Composting

I find composting very rewarding. Some people are put off by the idea as they dislike the smell. However, there are various odor-free compost collector canisters with effective filters that can be purchased online.

There is something special about returning organic matter back to the soil which produced it in the first place. Breaking up the compost and mixing it with fibrous matter (stalks and stems) and gravel, to help drainage and create fertile loam, is a lot of fun; and don't forget the health benefits of exchanging micro-bacteria while handling it.

Composting is much easier than most people realize. It can even be done in the small space of an apartment, to deliver nutrition to your house plants. This type of composting is called worm composting or vermicomposting. It's compact, uses basic and affordable materials, and can be done indoors or outdoors.[45] Keep in mind that it's often best to avoid adding meat or bones to your home or garden compost, as they attract pests and other wildlife.

---

45   U.S. Environmental Protection Agency, 2023. Composting at home. https://www.epa.gov/recycle/composting-home.

Another perk is having lots of free fertilizer! If you have no way of using it yourself, I'm sure you can give it to someone who can. Plenty of flowers, bushes, and trees would be thrilled to receive it.

If you have no space for composting yourself, utilize local municipal or community programs that collect or accept food scraps.[46]

If all this is not an option, electric composters will now shred and dehydrate your food scraps, turning them into soil overnight.[47]

Save Soil

Did you know that we would have to eat eight of today's oranges to derive the same nutritional value of one orange consumed in the 1920s? According to studies quoted by both Scientific American and The Organic Consumers Association, American produce has lost up to 80% of its nutrition since the 1950s.[48]

The reason our food is so much less nutritious than it used to be is because of what modern agriculture is doing to our planet and its soil. 52 % of agricultural soil is now degraded. Half of the topsoil, home to all the necessary micro-bacteria of our planet, has been lost in the last 150 years.[49]

We humans live an illusion of separateness. I am separate from you; my property is separate from yours; my country is not yours— but what about **our planet?**

The foundation of all life is Planet Earth. Through the Earth we are all interconnected; by the Earth we are all nurtured. We must realize that

---

[46] U.S. Environmental Protection Agency, 2023. Community composting. https://www.epa.gov/sustainable-management-food/community-composting.
[47] E.g. See www.mill.com.
[48] Corbley, 2023.
[49] United Nations University, 2015.

HOLISTIC EATING

> *Nature doesn't need people; people need nature.*

This is the recurring theme of a series of short films entitled *Nature is Speaking*, made by Conservation International. In particular, I urge you to watch *The Soil*, narrated by Edward Norton.

Dr. Wahls' extensive research on the amount of nutrition in modern foods leads her to recommend consuming nine cups of fruits and vegetables every day for what we need. When I share this with people, they are often surprised by the large amount recommended. Many people don't even consume that amount of vegetables in a month!

If we don't start caring for our soil, we will soon need to consume double that amount – eighteen cups a day! – to get the same nutritional benefit. One day, eating enough fruit and vegetables for our daily needs could become impossible. Although everyone will be affected, the poor will be most disadvantaged, as usual. Wealth will always find a way to appropriate higher quality, i.e. healthier organic food (with a higher price tag) for themselves. Keeping everybody nourished in an ever-growing population will become increasingly challenging without the foundation of a healthy soil.

"*When nature thrives, we thrive; when it falters, we falter*" is another quote from the powerful two-minute series, *Nature is Speaking*.

Just listen to Julia Roberts as the voice of Mother Nature:

> *I have fed species greater than you and I have starved species greater than you.*

We are not separate. We are one organism birthed by the same Mother Earth.

The Takeaways:

- Start cooking using the recipes in this or the previous chapter.
- Take pride in transforming your trash from inorganic to compostable matter.
- Start composting your organic leftovers and feed it to your plants or donate it to your local community farmers.
- See appendix for resources.

Chapter 8

From Healthcare to Self-Care

HEALTHCARE REVAMPED

Nobody can give us health; health is our responsibility. This has to be brought into our curriculum that every child in this country should learn how to generate health for himself, not wait for the healthcare system to help him later in his life, but he must become the main healthcare provider for himself.[50]

Sadhguru

You might have been paying for healthcare insurance all your life, expecting that you will be well taken care of if anything happens to you. Unfortunately, it doesn't work that way. The high insurance rates and deductibles that you have paid will not guarantee quality care.

The best guarantee you can have is to take things into your own hands and, as Sadhguru puts it, generate health for yourself. **You** are your best healthcare provider. You have many options, besides those which your insurance approves or disapproves of. Be open-minded, not controlled by the system, and don't let your choices be limited by what your insurance company tells you. Yes, it is unfortunate that we spend so much money on health insurance, which determines our choices and dictates our care, but if you see insurance for what it is, you can work your way around it. The system is corrupt, but the system doesn't define you and your health – you do.

Empowered, not Entitled

To begin with, we should realize it is better to feel empowered than to feel entitled. Because we pay a lot for our insurance, we expect a return on our investment. This expectation makes us feel entitled. The high insurance rates we've paid should surely give us the best quality care available. But however our investment turns out, there are still things that we can control. No matter which hospital, doctor or nurse is looking after us, expecting from others always poses a risk of disappointment. Rather, expect from yourself and accept those things you have no control over. By accepting, I don't mean agreeing. I disagree with the system, but I accept it for what it is. This allows me to determine my own choices within it in a clearer light.

The system **is** corrupt. We must acknowledge this but not make ourselves into victims. Feeling entitled is entangling, but feeling empowered is emancipating! We might have invested, but the return is beyond our control. If we feel entitled, our expectations hand the broken healthcare system the power to make us victims; but if we ourselves take charge, no one can make a victim out of us.

In my nursing practice, I encounter patients with differing attitudes. There are those – the entitled – who say, "*What can I get?*" There are others – the empowered – who say instead, "*What can I do?*" I can assure you that patients with a "*What can I do?*" attitude have a better recovery rate. Even the most incapacitated patients, if conscious, have choices.

Your attitude is a choice. It can either help you get healthy or make you sick.

Some patients and families I encounter complain about everything and anything. They write down the name of every professional that enters their hospital room; perhaps they have valid reasons to be mistrustful, but such an attitude often makes their experience worse. They create an environment conducive to sickness and disease, rather than to health and recovery. They arrive with expectations that are impossible to meet in today's dysfunctional healthcare system. While it is true that those with good insurance enter hospitals that are usually better equipped, our healthcare system is beset with problems everywhere. The current shortage of nurses and caregivers affects all hospitals and nursing homes, and is significantly lowering the quality of care that can be provided in them.

Healing Space

Looking for faults and blaming others is never going to bring an end to suffering. However, by bringing a positive attitude, patients and their families can transform the energy inside their hospital room in powerful ways. I have witnessed this transformation and what it can do, on many occasions. Families with empowered attitudes bring posters, pictures, and cards with inspirational messages; they bring music recordings or even instruments to play for their sick loved ones. They sing to them while they bath, moisturize, and massage their bodies. They create the most essential ingredient for the healing process: a healing space.

Exploring Different Options:

There is always more than one way of doing things. Our current healthcare system may present us with one particular way, but there are always others. We must not forget that. The moment we forget is the moment we allow ourselves to become limited.

Home Birth vs Hospital Birth

With the advancement of science and technology, the role of hospitals has expanded, and their number has grown exponentially. So has the number of hospital births; while home births, with the assistance of a midwife, have declined substantially. Safety during childbirth is naturally the number one priority, with the notion that hospitals are best at providing it. Fearful parents are reassured that a hospital birth is their best and only option, despite the financial strain that comes with it.

Yet even with this transition to giving birth in hospitals, our current statistics are dismal. Jacqueline Howard for CNN reported in 2023 that:

> The number of women who died of maternal causes in the United States rose to 1,205 in 2021, according to a report from the National Center for Health Statistics, released by the US Center for Disease Control and Prevention. That's a sharp increase from earlier: 658 in 2018, 754 in 2019, and 861 in 2020... The new report also notes significant racial disparities...In 2021, the rate for Black women was 69.9 deaths per 100,000 live births, which is 2.6 the rate for white women, at 26.6 per 100,000 [50]

When we research the safety of home births as opposed to hospital births, the data seems clear: hospital births are safer. It is important to note, though, that the statistics fail to accurately represent those healthy women, well cared for by a team of midwives and obstetricians, who successfully give birth at home. Although there are far fewer home births than hospital births, a significant number involve women with low socio-economic status, mental health problems, substance abuse, and who are victims of domestic violence. They receive no support or guidance; their life situation is high-risk to begin with.

A study published in "Obstetrics & Gynecology,"[51] which assessed violent deaths in pregnancy, reported that pregnancy-associated deaths accounted for more than 20% of all homicides of female victims reported to the CDC between 2008-2019. It concluded that mental health problems, substance use disorder and intimate partner violence often precede pregnancy-associated suicide and homicide.

Building bigger, better, and more beautiful hospitals with high-quality care, unobtainable to those who need it most, does not resolve the needs of our communities. It creates more disparity. We must look outside the hospitals and meet patients/mothers where they are, providing the care they require, instead of the type of care we want them to receive.

---

50 https://www.cnn.com/2023/03/16/health/maternal-deaths-increasing-nchs/index.html.
51 Modest et al., 2022.

Embracing Nature

Giving birth in a hospital has had a profound impact on the entire culture of childbearing. Hospitals are now chosen both for reasons of safety and for their ability to anesthetize birthing mothers. By eliminating labor pain, we have silenced nature and women's natural physiological processes. The obstetrician is now in charge of the entire process. A laboring mother who can't feel pain can't feel a contraction. She has no knowledge of when to push, or for how long, and feels no urgency to do so; she needs to be told and guided by the physician. This profound moment of female empowerment has been switched to one of total dependency.

My Birthing Experience

Home birth was unheard of when I had my children over 20 years ago. It required an intense argument with the insurance company to arrange coverage. I myself, as a young mother, gave birth in the hospital because I didn't realize other options existed.

I still remember the discomfort of the unfamiliar hospital environment. I felt scared and I felt a sense of inferiority. I remember the conflict between what was thought to be appropriate and my body's intuitive desire to take control. I remember the anger I felt during labor in trying to follow the doctor's directions, while forced to suppress my instinctive physiology.

For my first childbirth, I chose not to be anesthetized, nor did I have an epidural. I knew exactly when to push and what position would be best for me, and it certainly wasn't lying on my back with my feet up, spread open for the doctor's convenience. As he gave his orders, orders that failed to coincide with the immense urges of my labor pain screaming at me, had I been able, I honestly would have found a way to force him to stop.

Through my obstetrics (OB) rotation in nursing school, I have observed many births; women lying on their backs with their feet up in defiance of gravity, some in excruciating pain, exhausted from long hours of pushing.

Seeing their uncomfortable positions made me remember the distress of my own labor and the accumulating pressure in my lower back. I couldn't help but think how changing the laboring mother's position could bring her some much needed relief, and perhaps hasten the birth. How helpful it would be for the birthing mother to squat instead. Unfortunately, pain relief in the form of an epidural, as wonderful as it may feel, comes with its disadvantages: limited positioning is one. Numbness may prevent feeling pain, but it deprives the body of control.

Home Births

My dear friend Klaudia was able to withstand the objections of her insurance company and the fear-instilling voices of, "*What if something goes wrong?*" She gave birth at home and I was honored to be there. It was one of the most profound experiences of my life.

I watched her stay present, in her strong feminine energy, throughout this life-giving miracle. It was incredibly empowering to me as a woman. She embraced her nature and that vital part of herself that I had to suppress when I gave birth. She stayed connected to her body, guided by pain, observing, listening, reacting. Her connection was so sacred that no one dared interrupt it. She was cared for and supported by her loving husband, a wonderful midwife, her assistant, and myself. We were all a team who never forgot that she was in control and that we were only there to guide, assist and support her.

In emergency cases and in complicated births there is no doubt that hospitals are best equipped to cope. But what is also true in non-emergency cases is that there is no place like home. Instead of fearing the worst – what if something goes wrong? – why not support mothers to feel confident and empowered during childbirth? Why not give them the support they need to give birth safely in whichever way they choose?

Birthing Centers

Birthing centers are a great alternative for mothers who want to give birth naturally but who need extra support to feel safe and confident about their decisions. These provide a wonderful option, somewhere in between hospital and home. Located near a hospital, and managed by experienced midwives and trained personnel, birthing centers have all effective protocols in place, in case of emergency.

I'm glad these centers are making a comeback. Their number has more than doubled in the last decade and continues to grow. At present, there are more than 400 freestanding birth centers in the United States, covering 40 states and Washington DC.[52]

Sanitariums & Retreats

In the United States, the term "sanitarium" refers to a medical facility for long-term illness, used in the late-nineteenth and early-twentieth centuries predominantly to treat tuberculosis (TB) before the discovery of antibiotics. The word, sometimes spelled sanatorium or sanitorium, is derived from the Latin '*sanitas*' meaning health, or '*sano*' to heal. Before antibiotics, a regimen of rest, relaxation, good nutrition, clean mountain air, and exposure to sunlight offered patients the best chance of fighting off disease. Following the discovery of antibiotics, tuberculosis was no longer a significant public health threat, and in the United States and other countries, these facilities closed down. Antibiotics made their therapies seem unnecessary. In effect, scientific medicine and pharmaceuticals were triumphant, and alternative therapies were dismissed and forgotten.

Unlike in the United States, sanatoriums, as they are known in Europe, have never lost their usefulness. In Germany, Austria, Czech Republic, Poland, Russia, Hungary, Switzerland, Slovakia, Italy, Japan, Spain, and France, they evolved into wellness and rehabilitation retreats that are still highly valued

---

[52] AABC, 2023.

today. These health resorts often integrate modern medical treatments with natural therapies. They are located in scenic areas, creating a peaceful and healing environment similar to their historic counterparts.

They can be compared to spa resorts with medical personnel available for consultations. They may include rehabilitation services for patients recovering from surgeries, injuries or illnesses providing physical and occupational therapy; or may focus on chronic disease management with centers that specialize in respiratory, cardiovascular and metabolic disorders. Some are wellness retreats aimed at promoting health and wellbeing, which include massage therapy, hydrotherapy (like mineral water baths, thermal springs, cryotherapy, clay or mud baths, etc.), and mineral water inhalations. Indeed, some even have salt caves!

Others focus on psychiatric and mental health, providing a tranquil environment to treat or manage conditions such as stress, anxiety, depression, and addiction. They are often located away from cities, near forests, mountains or seas, and provide a variety of healthy foods accommodating different diets.

In the previously mentioned countries where sanatoriums still exist, they are affordable and, in most cases, can be covered by private insurance or governmental funding. For example, the Polish government provides funding for sanatorium treatments under the public healthcare system, primarily through the National Health Fund (Narodowy Fundusz Zdrowia, NFZ). To receive sanatorium treatment funded by the NFZ, you need a referral from a primary care physician or a specialist. The referral is then submitted to the NFZ, which evaluates the medical necessity and determines eligibility. If approved, you are placed on a waiting list. The wait time can vary depending on the type of treatment and the availability of spots at sanatoriums. It may even take as long as 3 years, but the stay may last between 21 to 28 days, and the services are available once every 18 months. If you prefer a specific sanatorium or quick access, you can always choose to pay for the treatment privately.

We are all still grateful for the discovery of antibiotics; but it is also true that a regimen of rest, relaxation, good nutrition, clean air and water, along with a safe healing space, boosts our immune system and is crucial in fighting off disease. Neither is a substitute for the other; instead, let's combine the two. When we use antibiotics or other medications, let's not forget the importance of our environment, our circumstances, and lifestyle. All of these are fundamental to health and healing.

Maintain a good relationship with yourself and cherish it, for that is most important of all. Learn to relax each day. Let go, stop pushing yourself, and create a healing environment for your body to regenerate and recover.

New advances and great discoveries continue to change and reshape lifestyles and humanity. We are constantly looking to improve and are finding new and often more straightforward ways to do so. Our modern lives may have become more efficient, but a vast number of people still suffer from stress. Enjoying more comfort than previous generations, ours is still prey to guilt, fear, anxiety, and depression.

Where did we go wrong? Perhaps life is not all about efficiency. Maybe life should be about balance – the balance between the old and the new; the balance between work and leisure. We should aim to achieve a balance of mind, body, and spirit and to live in harmony with nature and the world around us.

Spa Alternatives

As well as sanitariums, many other spa alternatives are available, including health and wellness retreats and educational workshops. One such place that transformed my life is the **Isha Institute of Inner-sciences-USA** (mentioned in Chapter Five under the section on meditation).

The Isha Institute restored my health and inner balance. There are now two locations within the US; one in Tennessee (that I attended) and the other newly established in California. The institute is open all year round to everyone. Set in a breathtaking mountain retreat, it offers guests:

...the essence of yogic science in its purest form, through classical yoga and meditation classes in powerfully energized spaces...[53]

It is mostly run by volunteers, making it very affordable and truly special. Everything there is done with care and devotion, ensuring you have the best experience.

I have visited the Isha Institute of Inner-Sciences multiple times, sometimes volunteering in their kitchen. There I learned not only how to prepare delicious vegetarian dishes, but also wonderful practices that continue to bring enormous meaning to my life.

One practice I have incorporated into my daily morning routine is Inner Engineering: *"...a comprehensive course for personal growth that brings about a shift in the way you perceive and experience your life, your work, and the world that you live in."*[54] Inner Engineering is a phenomenal experience for me that never ends. The ongoing practice continually expands my awareness and deepens my perception and understanding of life in profound ways.

Another healing opportunity that I learned about recently and that I have yet to experience is the **Dr. Joe Dispenza Retreat**. Through retreats, courses, and scientific studies, Dr. Joe Dispenza's method helps people replace fear-based thinking patterns with new limitless mindsets, providing evidence of profound physiological change by transforming our thought processes.

The Ann Wigmore Natural Health Institute is another retreat option, offering a "Living Foods Lifestyle" program that teaches optimal health through chlorophyll-rich and cultured foods. It is a two-week detoxification and cleansing program that includes a comprehensive education on the

---

53 Isha Institute of Inner-Sciences.
54 Isha Institute of Inner-Sciences.

benefits of raw, living foods. Diet, hands-on food preparation classes, detoxification techniques, and lifestyle practices are all aimed at rejuvenating health.

Another option to prioritize health and well-being is through silent retreats. One option is a ten-day silent retreat called **Vipassana meditation.** This ancient Buddhist practice, discovered by the Buddha 2,500 years ago, uses breath and body awareness to develop concentration and insight. Vipassana centers are located all over the world and are free of charge to those who seek to learn the practice.

I encourage you to explore for yourself any available opportunities and to pursue those which you personally find most rewarding and fulfilling. Don't wait for retirement to start taking care of yourself. Make the most of the time you have right now.

Earthing

> *Earthing (also known as grounding) refers to the discovery that bodily contact with the Earth's natural electric charge stabilizes physiology at the deepest levels, reduces inflammation, pain, and stress, improves blood flow, energy, and sleep, and generates greater well-being.*[55]

Being in touch with Mother Earth was once necessary for survival. 'Earthing' was an everyday experience, not a choice. Unfortunately, the more our lives change through advances in technology, the less grounded we become through contact with Mother Earth. These days we can live months, years – even most of our lives – never coming into contact with the soil. Not doing so is detrimental to our health. When we are looking for the causes of our diseases, we don't realize that some of the answers lie right beneath our feet.

---

55   Menigoz et al., 2020.

From house garage to work garage and back again, from parking lot to parking lot, from bedroom to office and to the front door to pick up the Amazon package we go, smartphone in hand, responding to texts every chance we get. So our lives go on like this, often without exposing ourselves to natural light. Modern innovations aimed at enhancing our comfort have distanced us from natural environments. Paradoxically, these are freeing and imprisoning us at the same time, yet we are too immersed to see it.

Since science became our primary way of understanding the world around us, we have now amassed data and proof which points to the health benefits of the way people used to live. For example, exposure to natural light within the first ten minutes of waking stimulates the hormones responsible for wakefulness throughout the day. Exposure to blue light during the evenings and late at night, often caused by electronic devices, disrupts our sleep cycles.

One way to know this is to study science; another is to explore and find out for yourself. To do this, get out of your daily routine. Leave all your devices behind and go outside; get off the pavement and into the grass. Walk barefoot. Hug trees. Make snowballs. So what if your clothes get dirty? It's healthy for you!

Mindfulness Practice

Most importantly, pay attention. Each time you get stuck in a thought, acknowledge the thought but start paying attention to your surroundings.

The mind will be less likely to take over when we do something out of the ordinary. Removing ourselves from our comfort zone is an excellent practice because it helps us pay full attention to what we're doing. Practice mindfulness for 30 minutes a day and notice the changes in how you feel. Ignore feelings of resistance. Reluctance to change is responsible for the self-imprisoning that we habitually do. Escape outside and be free; the discomfort will pass and new feelings of gratitude and happiness will arise.

The Takeaways:

- Turn your home into a healing space. Use natural incense or essential oils to make it smell beautiful.
- Rub oils onto your skin, appreciating your body.
- Soak in the bath using bath salts like eucalyptus, clove, and peppermint.
- Practice Earthing every day by lying down on the grass for at least a few minutes (use a towel or a blanket if necessary). Take a walk in silence. Walk barefoot. Breathe in the fresh air. Enjoy nature.

Chapter 9

Eliminating Toxins

Toxic Load

Toxic load is the total amount of harmful substances accumulated in the body over time. Lowering our toxic load is essential for staying healthy. As we have already seen, there are many toxic substances in our food, but a lot are also found in cosmetics and cleaning supplies. Take a field trip around your living space and examine all the products you use. Look at their ingredients – are they even listed? If not, or if the list is a long one with lots of chemical materials formulated in a laboratory, substitute the product with something natural.

In selecting cosmetics such as make-up, we look for the right color, easy application, and the ability to look fresh without needing to reapply it throughout the day or through the evening. When we search for creams, we like them to smell nice, be compatible with our skin type, and have the right consistency. With soaps and shampoos, we look for products that will make a lather to take off dirt and grease without leaving our skin and hair dry and damaged; we also want them to have a great smell, leaving us feeling clean and refreshed.

But when looking for these desirable qualities in our products, do we think about the chemical processes involved? Many ground-breaking discoveries in chemistry are applied in the manufacture of cosmetics. We now have fancy thickeners, softeners, solvents, moisture carriers, surfactants, emulsifiers, and foaming agents that make our cosmetics just the way we like them. A lot of knowledge, work, and experimentation goes into making these lavish and sophisticated smells happen for us.

As we spend more time indoors using more abrasive, and therefore more toxic, substances to keep clean, we spend much less time outdoors getting dirty exploring the tangible world. Our daily surroundings in our homes and at the workplace are cleaner than at any previous time in our history. The cleaner we live, the more fixated on cleanliness we become, disinfecting everything to the point of causing harm. Nowadays we are much less likely to break a sweat, but more inclined to use harsh chemicals in case we do.

All these fancy chemical products do not come without a price to our overall health. We may not sweat or smell bad, or have greasy hair, but our toxic load has risen exponentially. As we deny and stop our body's natural processes, we confuse our immune system. It is no longer capable of distinguishing its own natural processes from synthetic and dangerously harmful ones.

Harmful Substances in Cosmetics

Antimicrobial and antifungal agents like parabens, formaldehyde donors and triclosan are some of the harmful ingredients found in the personal care products we use every day. They are present in cosmetics, soaps, detergents and toothpaste.

Parabens, for example, are a group of synthetic preservatives that prevent the growth of bacteria, mold, and yeast, thereby extending product shelf life. There have been concerns about their potential link to hormone disruption by their ability to mimic estrogen in the body. These substances accumulate in, and are harmful to, aquatic life and other organisms.[56]

Other potentially harmful ingredients are surfactants, emulsifiers, and foaming agents. Take surfactants, for example. Surfactants lower the surface tension of liquids, making them easier to mix with water and work into a foam. Some surfactants commonly used in shampoos, toothpaste, soaps, and cleansers contain sulfates. The drawback with sulfates is that they are too effective at cleaning. In shampoos, they may strip away too much moisture, leaving hair dry and unhealthy. They may also make the scalp dry and prone to irritation.

When inspecting ingredient labels, it is important to note that some chemicals are not inherently harmful, but their derivatives or certain uses can raise concerns.

---

56 Halden et al., 2017.

Ethanolamine and ethoxylated compounds are chemicals used in products like shampoos, soaps, and cleaners. They are also used in some industrial processes. These chemicals are useful because they can act as surfactants, emulsifiers, solubilizers, conditioning agents, and more.

To make these chemicals, manufacturers react ethylene oxide with other substances like alcohols or phenols. This reaction changes the properties of the original substances. It can make them more soluble in water or better at reducing surface tension.

Some ethanolamine derivatives may pose risks when exposed to certain conditions. For example, when ethanolamines react with certain other chemicals, they form nitrosamines. One form of nitrosamine is a potent carcinogen and has been linked to various cancers. Readily absorbed through the skin, it accumulates in the liver, bladder, and other organs. Studies have also linked nitrosamines to developmental or reproductive toxicity, immunotoxicity, neurotoxicity, and systemic toxicity.[57]

Nitrosamines are not listed on the label since they may be formed by reactions between the other ingredients. Consumers cannot easily tell which products contain them. Avoid products with DEA, TEA, and other ethanolamine compounds since these contribute to nitrosamine formation.

Thickeners, Softeners, Solvents, and Moisture Carriers

Propylene Glycol (PEG) is a petroleum-based synthetic organic compound that serves as a thickener, softener, solvent, and moisture carrier. Ethylene oxide plays a key role in their production, and PEG is likely to become contaminated with it, as well as with the chemical compound known as 1,4-dioxane; both are carcinogens.[58]

---

57 Safe Cosmetics, n.d.
58 FDA, 2022.

Unfortunately, these are just a few harmful chemicals among many more. If I were to make a list of all compounds to avoid in cosmetics/makeup, it would be nearly impossible to follow. The list would be so long, with so many long names similar to each other, it would be very confusing. In addition, one molecular change to a compound results in a name change, making it difficult to keep up with the ongoing updates. However, for a simplified shoppers guide to help avoid the "dirty dozen" found in cosmetics, visit davidsuzuki.org (https://davidsuzuki.org/living-green/dirty-dozen-cosmetic-chemicals-avoid/)[59]

Simple Ingredients

We don't need to use such harsh chemicals to keep ourselves clean. Many people have office jobs and barely spend any time outside, yet our hygiene practices have reached unprecedented levels. Most of the time simple ingredients will do just fine. For instance, I like to use Dr. Bronner's 18-in-1 uses, Pure-Castile hemp soap (scented with organic essential oils).

Should you get frustrated with your body for rejecting something you used or ate, remember that its reaction is there to communicate danger and to protect you. Trusting and respecting my body has been a most gratifying experience for me. I once went to a sales presentation on anti-aging creams. Although I am a person interested only in natural products, even I was lured into buying the lab-made anti-aging collection that was supposed to make me look young and beautiful. Instead, I got an allergic reaction with hives all over my face – just in time for Christmas!

Although I was annoyed, I was also grateful for my body speaking to me in such a way. Even if I get lazy and don't feel like researching all the confusing product ingredients, my body often makes sure I know right away. My body can know instantaneously what would take hours to learn and understand; it saves me from diseases. All I must do is pay attention. As long as my mind and body stay integrated, understanding each other, I can stay out of trouble.

---

59 Web address correct at time of publication: 2025.

Homemade Natural Substitutes

Fancy, expensive, and often toxic products purchased at the store can be substituted with more affordable versions made at home from natural, non-toxic ingredients and essential oils. Not only are homemade products less abrasive, but they are also pleasant to make. Essential oils, baking soda and vinegar are the basis for many home-made cleaning agents. Moisturizers, as well as face and hair masks, are easy to make yourself using essential oils, coconut oil and 100% aloe vera gel. Using essential oil in diffusers, nebulizers, sprays, and even car fresheners is a healthy, non-toxic way to make the space around you smell great. It assures that you're inhaling therapeutic molecules instead of toxins. Roll-ons and body sprays will make you smell fresh throughout the day while stimulating your olfactory nerves, sending powerful signals throughout your central nervous system. Aromatherapy has been proven to restore the olfactory sensation after viral infections like COVID-19.[60] I use a baby blender to mix them and store them in dark glass jars or glass bottles to protect them from light and preserve their efficacy, as they will not keep for long otherwise. I recommend Dr. Keesha's DIY Autoimmune Home Detox: *Healing from the Inside Out*, which includes many cleaning and beauty products you can make at home.

---

60   Abalo-Lojo et al., 2023.

Here are some of my favorite home-made recipes.[61]

HOMEMADE MULTI-SURFACE CLEANING SPRAY

Ingredients:

- 1 cup distilled water
- 1/2 cup white vinegar
- 10 drops tea tree essential oil
- 10 drops lemon essential oil
- 10 drops sweet orange essential oil
- Reusable spray bottle

Directions:

1. In a clean spray bottle, combine the distilled water, white vinegar, and essential oils.
2. Secure the spray top and give the bottle a gentle shake to mix the ingredients thoroughly.
3. Before each use, give the bottle a light shake to ensure the oils are well-distributed.
4. To use, simply spray the cleaning solution directly onto countertops, bathroom surfaces, sinks, and most floor types. Always test a small, inconspicuous area first to ensure the solution won't cause any discoloration or damage.
5. Allow the solution to sit for a few moments, then wipe clean with a soft, lint-free cloth or paper towel.

Notes:

The combination of vinegar, tea tree oil, lemon, and sweet orange essential oils creates a natural, fresh-scented cleaner with antimicrobial properties.

---

61 Reproduced here by the kind permission of Dr. Keesha.

HEALTHCARE REVAMPED

Adjust the essential oil quantities to suit your preferred scent strength.

Store the spray bottle out of direct sunlight and away from heat sources.

Discard any unused portion after a few months and make a fresh batch for optimal potency.

HOMEMADE DEODORANT

Ingredients:

- 3 tablespoons coconut oil
- 3 tablespoons baking soda
- 2 tablespoons Shea butter
- 2 tablespoons arrowroot powder
- ½ tablespoon beeswax
- 1 tablespoon jojoba
- 1 tablespoon bentonite clay
- ½ tablespoon magnesium hydroxide
- 25 to 30 drops of essential oils (Clary sage, lavender bergamot, and cypress)

Instructions:

1. Combine shea butter, beeswax, and coconut oil in an open glass jar and place in a small saucepan of water over medium heat. Allowed to sit until the wax, shea butter and coconut oil are completely melted.
2. Remove from heat and add the rest of the ingredients: baking soda, arrowroot, Jojoba oil, bentonite clay, magnesium hydroxide, and essential oils.
3. Mix well. Allow it to sit in a jar until cool and then cover it to store.
4. Applied to underarms as needed.

EASY COCONUT OIL DEODORANT

Ingredients:

- 6 tablespoons coconut oil
- 1/4 cup baking soda
- 1/4 cup arrowroot powder
- Essential oil as desired (Clary sage, lavender, bergamot, cypress)

Instructions:

1. Mix the baking soda and arrowroot together and add in softened coconut oil, steering into a smooth. Add essential oils as desired.
2. Store in a small jar or stick deodorant dispenser and apply under arms as needed.

SUPER DRY MEN'S DEODORANT

Ingredients:

- 1/4 cup arrowroot powder
- 3 tablespoons baking soda
- 2 tablespoons diatomaceous earth or bentonite clay
- 6 tablespoons coconut oil
- 1.5 tablespoons beeswax palettes
- 8 drops orange essential oil
- 18 drops cypress essential oil
- 8 drops frankincense essential oil
- Other essential oil options:
- Clove, cinnamon, orange
- Cypress, juniper Berry
- Bergamot, cedarwood
- Sandalwood, patchouli
- Sweet orange, patchouli
- Lemon, fir needle

Instructions:

1. In a Mason jar, add the beeswax and coconut oil.
2. Place the jar in a pot with several inches of water in it, and heat over medium-high heat until melted.
3. Add the remaining ingredients and stir until combined.
4. Pour contents into a small glass jar or stick deodorant dispenser and cool.
5. Use underarms as needed.

HOMEMADE HAND SANITIZER

Ingredients:

- 3 tablespoons aloe Vera gel
- 1 tablespoon filtered water
- 5 drops tea tree essential oil
- 5 drops lavender essential oil
- 1 teaspoon vitamin E
- 1 teaspoon vitamin C

Instructions:

1. Combine all ingredients together into a well blended.
2. Pour into squeeze bottle.
3. Use as needed directly on hands and do not rinse.

ALL-NATURAL FACIAL MOISTURIZER

Ingredients:

- 3 oz organic unrefined melted coconut oil
- 1 oz organic unrefined melted Shea butter
- 1 oz organic pure aloe Vera gel
- 1 oz organic Jojoba oil
- 1 oz emu oil
- 20 drops Hyaluronic Acid
- 10 drops vitamin E oil
- 10 drops vitamin C oil
- 10 drops rosehip seed oil
- 10 drops carrot seed oil
- 10 drops frankincense essential oil
- 10 drops sandalwood essential oil
- 10 drops lavender essential oil

Instructions:

1. Blend all ingredients in a blender until creamy.
2. Pour contents into a glass jar with a tight-fitting lid.
3. Applied to clean, dry face every morning and bedtime.

HOMEMADE SUN PROTECTORS

Making homemade sunscreen is fun, and will allow you to avoid using harmful chemicals. Chemicals found in commercial sunscreens are oxybenzone (benzophenone-3), octinoxate (ethylhexyl methoxycinnamate), homosalate, octocrylene, avobenzone, parabens (like methylparaben, or propylparaben) and triclosan. A safer alternative is using sunscreens with mineral-based active ingredients like zinc oxide, or titanium dioxide.

But before you start using your homemade natural sunscreen, it is important you know how to use them correctly, to stay safe while bathing in the sun. SPF stands for Sun Protection Factor and it is a numerical estimate of how well a product protects your skin from ultraviolet B (UVB) rays. Unlike sunscreens that absorb UV radiation, sunblocks are products designed to deflect and block those harmful rays by forming a physical barrier on the surface of the skin. It is that white coating of the sunscreen that provides the protective layer blocking the sun's rays.

Dermatologists usually recommend SPF 30 sunscreen at the very least. Natural sunscreens use active ingredients from plants to coat the skin and reflect UV rays, making it challenging to accurately estimate the exact SPF of a homemade sun protector. Always be mindful of your skin type, how easily you burn, how long you are out in the sun, and the intensity of its rays, depending on the region and the time of the day. I live in a region where the sun is low and its rays less powerful than in Hawaii, so my homemade sunscreen is sufficient most of the time. But if I were to travel to say Hawaii or Greece, and spend most of my time on a sailing boat, I would want to purchase a sunscreen that would guarantee the recommended protection, and be water resistant.

When buying sunscreen look for one approved under Hawaii's Sunscreen Law (Act 104), which bans the sale and distribution of sunscreens containing the above-mentioned oxybenzone, and octinoxate. These chemicals have been found to cause coral bleaching, to damage coral DNA and disrupt the growth and reproduction of coral and other marine life.[62] Instead, you

---

[62] Downs, 2014.

can buy 100% mineral-based sunscreen containing zinc oxide or titanium dioxide. These ingredients are considered safe for marine environments and provide effective broad-spectrum protection against UV radiation.

Here are my 2 favorite sunscreen recipes:

DR KEESHA'S HOMEMADE SUNSCREEN RECIPE[63]

Ingredients:

- Half a cup Jojoba oil (may use almond or olive also)
- 1/4 cup coconut oil (natural SPF 4)
- 1/4 cup beeswax
- 2 tablespoons zinc oxide (high-quality nano zinc oxide purchased from reputable suppliers who provide information on particle size, purity, and safety and be careful not to inhale the powder)
- 1 teaspoon emu oil
- 1 teaspoon vitamin E serum
- 1 teaspoon carrot seed oil
- 2 tablespoons Shea butter (natural SPF 4 to 15)

Instructions:

1. Combine all but the zinc oxide in a quart-sized Mason jar.
2. Place in a pan of water and heat over medium heat. Stir periodically until all the ingredients are melted.
3. Carefully add the zinc oxide and stir well ensuring even distribution.
4. Pour into small glass jars with lids. Stir with a toothpick occasionally as it cools to make sure the zinc oxide is blended in well.

Store in the refrigerator or in a cool dark place to maintain stability and effectiveness.

---

63 Reproduced here by the kind permission of Dr. Keesha.

HOMEMADE SUNSCREEN WITH ALOE VERA AND COCONUT OIL [64]

Ingredients

- 1/4 cup coconut oil (has an SPF of 7)
- 2 (or more) tbsp. powdered zinc oxide
- 1/4 cup pure aloe vera gel (must be 50 percent or higher)
- 25 drops walnut extract oil for scent and an added SPF boost
- 1 cup (or less) shea butter for a spreadable consistency

Instructions

1. Combine all ingredients, except the zinc oxide and aloe vera gel, in a medium saucepan. Let the shea butter and oils melt together at medium heat.
2. Let cool for several minutes before stirring in aloe vera gel.
3. Cool completely before adding zinc oxide. Mix well to make sure the zinc oxide is distributed throughout. You may want to add some beeswax or another waxy substance for a stickier consistency.

Store in a glass jar, and keep in a cool, dry place until you're ready to use.

---

[64] Watson, 2019.

Essential Oils

There is a lot to know about essential oils and how to choose the best brands out there. Their therapeutic use for the treatment and management of many chronic illnesses, including insomnia, low libido, fibromyalgia, COPD, cancer, anxiety, depression, diabetes and more is well worth the research.[65] Spend some time and empower yourself by learning about them. See the appendix for resources.

Some of my favorite resources on the use of essential oils and their healing properties (with thousands of recipes) are **naturallivingfamily.com** and **aromatics.com**[66]

Fungal Infections

Fungal infections like *Candida*, responsible for yeast infections, and *Malassezia* yeast, which causes tinea versicolor (discolored patches on the skin, often on the trunk and shoulders) are becoming more common and can be very difficult to get rid of. They may go away for a while after the use of antifungal creams, only to come back again. Fungi feed on sugar and prefer a slightly acidic environment. Changing from an acidic diet, containing high amounts of sugar, grains and dairy, to a more alkaline, high-fiber diet is crucial for achieving long-term results. Essential oils, tea tree in particular, are a wonderful alternative to antifungal creams. In addition, tea tree oil is also an effective natural remedy for various skin issues such as minor cuts and insect bites.

Here is my favorite DIY antifungal and anti-inflammatory tea tree oil ointment recipe:

---

65 Zielinski, 2022.
66 Website addresses correct at time of publication: 2024.

TEA TREE OIL OINTMENT

Ingredients:

- 1/4 cup coconut oil (or another carrier oil such as castor, olive or jojoba oil)
- 1/4 cup beeswax pellets (to give the ointment a solid consistency)
- 10-20 drops tea tree essential oil (adjust based on desired potency)
- Optional: 5-10 drops of other essential oils, like lavender or eucalyptus for added benefits and fragrance

Equipment:

- Double boiler (or a heatproof bowl and a pot)
- Stirring utensil (like a spoon or wooden stick)
- Small, clean jars or tins for storing the ointment

Instructions:

1. **Prepare the Double Boiler:** If you don't have a double boiler, you can create one by placing a heatproof bowl over a pot of simmering water. Ensure the bottom of the bowl doesn't touch the water.
2. **Melt the Beeswax:** Add the beeswax pellets to the double boiler. Stir occasionally until the beeswax is completely melted.
3. **Add the Carrier Oil:** Once the beeswax is melted, add the coconut oil (or your chosen carrier oil) to the mixture. Stir well, until both the beeswax and oil are fully combined and melted together.
4. **Remove from Heat:** Carefully remove the mixture from heat once the beeswax and carrier oil are thoroughly mixed.
5. **Add Tea Tree Oil:** Allow the mixture to cool slightly, but not harden. Add 10-20 drops of tea tree essential oil, depending on the desired strength. If using additional essential oils, add them at this stage too. Stir well to ensure they are evenly distributed.

ELIMINATING TOXINS

6. Pour into Containers: Pour the mixture into small, clean jars or tins. Let it cool and solidify at room temperature. You can place the containers in the refrigerator to speed up the cooling process, if desired.
7. Label and Store: Label the containers with the date and contents. Store the ointment in a cool, dark place to prolong its shelf life. It should last for several months.

Good Rule to Follow

Overall, a good rule to follow about skin applications is: if it's edible, it's safe to put on your skin. The only negative is that natural products don't last as long as synthetic ones. But remember, the toxins that make them last longer are what you're trying to avoid anyway. Most of the products you create yourself have to be made fresh in small amounts, or kept in the refrigerator.

Makeup

When people search for toxic products in their homes, makeup can be easily overlooked. But don't be fooled – it often makes the list of the most dangerous. In addition to known carcinogens, all sorts of nasty stuff have been discovered in makeup: heavy metals like lead and mercury, super glue, and even animal feces. One reason? – much of it is counterfeited. It may look like the real thing, yet be an illegal imitation of a reputable brand.[67] Double-check the source, and if the cheap price sounds too good to be true, it most likely is.

Even the most reputable brands are not safe. A 2023 analysis of 50 random facial cosmetics commercially available in the European Union revealed the presence of potentially carcinogenic substances.[68] When purchasing makeup, look for clean and sustainable brands that contain a list of ingredients. Don't hesitate to reach out to the merchant with any questions or concerns you have, before you buy their product. They should be able to back up their claims and provide information about their sourcing, sustainability, and ingredients.

Or you might want to have some fun and make your own instead!

---

67   Rivo, 2019.
68   Balwierz et al., 2023.

HOMEMADE BLUSH RECIPE[69]

Ingredients:

- ½ teaspoon arrowroot powder
- ½ teaspoon organic cocoa powder
- ½ teaspoon hibiscus powder
- Optional: mica for shimmer (natural, cosmetic-grade)
- Air-tight container for storage

Instructions:

You will need to play with ratios as the amount used will vary by person according to your desired shade. Start with half a teaspoon of arrowroot powder and add the hibiscus and the cocoa powder to darken as desired, testing on your inner arm as you go. You can add a little mica if you want a fairy shimmer. Store in a glass jar with a lid.

A Good Rule to Follow:

If bugs, mold, and bacteria are quick to grow in a product, it often reflects its good quality and non-toxicity. If they like it, it means that it's not toxic to them and won't be harmful to you. Rather be alarmed when products you buy sit in your cupboards or your refrigerator for months without deteriorating. Chances are, not even bacteria want to eat them!

---

69 Reproduced here by the kind permission of Dr. Keesha.

Food Products

If bacteria and mold don't even want to touch a food product, how will the bacteria in your gut react when you consume it? If your gut bacteria get fed with toxic foods, a lot of them will be destroyed and this creates a microbiome imbalance within your body. Some bacterial colonies become smaller or die off completely; others take over to the point of becoming unhealthy pathogens.

Your diet is what feeds these tiny organisms living inside you; their life is essential to your life. More and more studies show that a well-balanced and diverse microbiome is a prerequisite for good health. Without bacteria to protect us, we get sick. Remember this whenever you begin to compulsively disinfect everywhere.

Pesticides

If you have any experience in gardening or growing your own food, you know that organic non-sprayed fruits and vegetables taste much better than what is sold at the stores. You also know how difficult it is to keep pests away. With the help of the internet, you can research and find homemade remedies in place of toxic pesticides. Sprays with just the right concentration of vinegar, salt or citric acid may deter pests without harming your plants or the environment.

For those seeking inspiration in the art of gardening and farming, I highly recommend watching one of my favorite movies, *The Biggest Little Farm* (2019), directed by John Chester. It portrays a couple who work together to produce a healthy ecosystem on their organic sustainable farm, with the most amazing results. Via a journey of hard work, they discover many secrets of nature. Their accomplishment is remarkable and the movie is a true masterpiece.

Nothing Fantastic About Too Much Plastic

In the field of human discovery, there seems to be a common theme. Discovering new products often comes with the significant advantage of simplifying our lives, only to complicate them further in the long run. The more sophisticated our discoveries, the more complex their consequences. Mass production and genetic modifications of food were expected to end world hunger. Instead, we are depleting the soil of necessary nutrients and may face hunger on a much grander scale in the future. The most promising ideas and inventions might, over time, reveal themselves to be harmful.

Microplastic

Plastic is one of these breakthrough inventions. Because of the endless opportunities introduced by plastic, it started to be used for everything and anything. As with asbestos, its toxicity was not realized at first. However, there are now many scientific studies that reveal the harmful toxins discovered in plastic such as bisphenol A (BPA), phthalates and polychlorinated biphenyls (PCB), with others still awaiting scientific investigation. It turns out that all this plastic accumulates in our bodies in the form of microplastic. Measuring microplastic deposition in human organs and blood is complex, but as our technical skills improve new data emerges.

Microplastics have been detected in various human body parts and fluids, such as the placenta, meconium, breast milk, lungs, intestines, liver, heart, cardiovascular system, blood, urine and cerebrovascular fluid, according to recent spectroscopy and spectrometry studies. Mounting research indicates that microplastics can have worrying effects on human cells, primarily through oxidative stress, inflammation and fibrosis.[70]

Once plastic gets inside our bodies, it's nearly impossible to get out. We can't avoid plastic, because we use so much of it. Most of our environment, the

---

70   La Porta, E., et al. (2023). Microplastics and kidneys. *Int J Mol Sci, 24*(18), 14391.

air we breathe, the food we eat, and the water we drink, is now contaminated with it. Plastic dispersion and its negative consequences on our health have become a significant concern.

Plastic waste dispersing into the environment has emerged as a major challenge facing humanity. Microplastics have spread everywhere, leading to daily human exposure through inhaling or ingesting these tiny plastic particles.

Xenoestrogens

While hormone disruptors like xenoestrogens are not plastics, certain types of plastics and plastic-related chemicals like BPA and phthalates are known to contain or release xenoestrogens. These mimic hormones and therefore disrupt our endocrine system – the network of glands that secrete hormones directly into the bloodstream. More research is in progress assessing its link to other diseases, including cancer.

Bisphenol A (BPA)

Bisphenol A (BPA) is one of the plastic-related chemicals known to contain or release xenoestrogens. It is found in the polycarbonate plastics and epoxy resins that are often used in food and beverage containers, water bottles and the lining of metal cans. It can leach from these containers into our food and drinks, especially when heated.[71] BPA has been linked to various health problems, including reproductive issues, developmental problems in children and an increased risk of certain cancers.[72]

Phthalates

Phthalates are used as plasticizers to make plastics like PVC more flexible and durable. They are found in products such as toys, food packaging,

---

71 National Institute of Environmental Health Sciences. (n.d.). Bisphenol A (BPA).
72 Cimmino, I., et al, 2020. Potential mechanisms of BPA contributing to human disease.

medical devices and personal care products. Phthalates can leach out of products and be ingested, inhaled or absorbed through the skin. They are associated with reproductive and developmental problems, hormone disruption and other health issues.[73]

Polychlorinated Biphenyls (PCB's)[74]

Although no longer manufactured in many countries, polychlorinated biphenyls (PCBs) were previously used in various industrial applications. For example, they served as plasticizers in paints and plastics, as well as in electrical equipment. PCBs are persistent organic pollutants that accumulate in the environment and food chain. This leads to adverse health effects like cancer, suppressed immune systems, and disruption of the endocrine system.

Plastic Resin Codes, Types, and Common Uses:

Plastic products are labeled with resin identification codes or recycling symbols to indicate the type of plastic used. Some plastics pose lower risks of leaching harmful chemicals into food or the environment compared to others.

---

73   Wang, Y., & Qian, H., 2021. Phthalates and their impacts on human health.
74   Montano, L., et al., 2022. PCBs in the environment: Effects on health and fertility.

Table:

Plastic Code	Abbreviation	Plastic Name	Common Uses
#1	PEPTE or PET	Polyethylene Terephthalate	Water and soda bottles, food containers, polyester clothing
#2	HDPE	High-Density Polyethylene	Milk jugs, detergent bottles, plastic bags, some toys
#3	PVC	Polyvinyl Chloride	Plastic bags, shrink wrap, flexible packaging
#4	LDPE	Low-density Polyethylene	Pipes, vinyl siding, window frames, flooring materials
#5	PP	Polypropylene	Food containers, bottle caps, automotive parts
#6	PS	Polystyrene	Disposable cups, takeout containers, packaging materials
#7	Other	Miscellaneous Plastic	Includes polycarbonate (CDs, eyeglasses), bioplastics, and other specialized materials

Based on current knowledge, plastics coded #2 (HDPE), #4 (LDPE) and #5 (PP) are considered among the safer options for use. However, it's important to note that the production process for all plastics is highly toxic to the environment. Anything that harms our environment ultimately affects human health as well, so I encourage you to limit your use of plastic.

Trash Problem

Our trash is growing in unmanageable proportions. The United States generates a huge amount of waste annually 268 million tons. A significant portion, 140 million tons, ends up in landfills every year. On average, each American throws away 4.5 pounds of trash daily.[75] It floats in our seas and permeates our waters. The indiscriminate presence of plastic in our oceans exacts a heavy toll, claiming the lives of thousands of seabirds, sea turtles, seals, and other marine creatures annually when they eat it or get entangled by it.[76] They mistake it for food and die as a result. Fish also ingest microplastics, and since they are part of our food chain, we ingest microplastics too when we eat fish.

We must strive to limit the use of plastic and become far more mindful of how we use it. New Jersey, for example, has installed restrictions on single-use plastic bags and styrofoam-like products at all grocery stores, restaurants, and other businesses. The plastic bag ban implemented from May through December 2022 prevented approximately 5 billion plastic bags from entering the waste stream, according to typical store usage estimates.[77]

Since plastic is used for so many things that make our lives convenient, I know how challenging it is to avoid it, but it's not impossible. New Jersey has produced such incredible results in a short time, and I hope more states will follow suit; but for now, we must ban plastic ourselves. Carry reusable shopping bags and say no when offered a plastic one. Use washable, organic cotton mesh bags for groceries and shop at stores where that's possible, rather than at stores where everything is prepackaged. We should limit our eating out, and when we do, always use our own stainless steel coffee cup or water bottle.

Being mindful of our plastic use and the trash we ourselves produce is part of the practice of awareness. We should aim to develop new and healthy

---

75 McDonald, 2023.
76 Center for Biological Diversity, 2024.
77 Rodas, 2023.

ways to avoid plastic. These can be fun. Most importantly, don't microwave food in plastic containers, and never microwave anything covered in plastic wrap; take it out of the container or wrapping, and put it on a ceramic plate.

Recycling

The idea of collecting and processing materials that would otherwise be discarded as waste, and transforming them into new products, is brilliant. Recycling is meant to conserve resources, reduce landfills, save energy and mitigate pollution. So why is it that out of the 46 million tons of plastic waste generated annually in the US, only 5% to 6% is currently recycled, a significant decline from the previous estimate of nearly 9%.[78]

Things are much more complicated than we imagine. For starters, the material must be cleaned before melting or shredding. If the melted or shredded material is contaminated with waste, this alters its chemical structure and it can no longer be recycled. When this happens the entire mix must be discarded. Cleansing trash from organic contaminants such as food waste and then sorting and separating it according to its type paper, glass, metal or plastic – is critical to successful recycling. In addition, plastic requires further sorting into its different classifications – see the table above. All this preparatory work is time-consuming and requires a lot of manpower, making the process expensive.

Furthermore, some trash like electronics must be dismantled before its parts can be segregated. Others are made from different types of mixed materials that cannot be separated, things such as toothbrushes, disposable razors, pens, and markers. Undergoing the melting process itself changes the chemical structure of the materials being recycled, affecting their quality and strength; often new materials need to be added to regain their original durability. Contaminating fumes are also produced during this process, which pollute the environment further and may negate the benefits of recycling.

---

78   Kummer, 2022.

The waste management resources between municipalities differ significantly, meaning that the recycling processes are inconsistent across different states, townships, and villages. These inconsistencies make recycling laws difficult to standardize and enforce. Residents find them hard to keep up with and implement. For these reasons, there is still much confusion and misinformation within the general public on the subject of waste management and recycling.

Wish-cycling

Just because a product says recyclable on it, does not mean it gets recycled. Tossing it into a recycling bin doesn't guarantee it will be recycled. And just because the recycle bins are collected by a specific waste management team, that does not mean that all of them will get recycled.

Most of us use plastic, thinking that it will get recycled, but in reality, the chance for that water bottle, milk jug, plate, utensil, toy, or toothbrush to get a second life is slim. It is more likely to make its way onto a cargo ship and travel across the border to a different country.

Currently, manufacturing a product using new material is less expensive than using recycled material. Since using new material is easier, cheaper in the short term, and produces consistent quality, we generate more trash than we can handle, let alone properly recycle. We simply can't keep up.

In 2023 around 37% of US plastic waste was exported to other countries. In previous years it was shipped to China, but after China's retreat from the global scrap plastic trade, it is now exported to other countries like Canada, Mexico, India, Malaysia, and Vietnam.[79]

We must remember that just because the waste we produce gets picked up by the waste management company each week, and we don't have to deal with it anymore, does not mean that the issue is resolved.

---

79 Resource Recycling, 2024.

Other commonly used hard-to-recycle items that often end up in landfills are: umbrellas, plastic tableware, and utensils that are often contaminated with food, balloons, ceramics, pottery, coffee pods like K-cups, CDs, DVDs, and plastic bags.

"Sacred Economics"

According to American public speaker, teacher, and author Charles Eisenstein in his groundbreaking book *Sacred Economics: Money, Gift & Society in the Age of Transition*,80 we must shift from looking only at the market value of a product to considering its environmental impact and sustainability. Incorporating the environmental and social cost of a product into its price can make recycled materials more economically viable.

Implementing policies that reward recycling and the use of recycled materials, such as subsidies, tax breaks, and other regulatory support, makes recycling more competitive. For example, in Hawaii and a few other states, each plastic or glass bottle and aluminum can has a stated amount of value when returned to the drop-off centers. You get paid for recycling your trash. In some stores you get a discount or financial credit for declining a bag or bringing your own. In Germany carry-out coffee is not sold in disposable plastic cups but in a mug, costing you an extra fee which is credited back with your next purchase. In Costa Rica and Europe straws are often made from paper. Holding producers accountable for the lifecycle of their products can drive innovation in sustainable design and recycling.

Reusing and repurposing items becomes more common in a culture that values sharing over owning. We must shift from associating wealth and happiness with owning and having. Instead, we should take pleasure in caring for our world through the experience of sharing, giving and reusing. Adopting a minimalist lifestyle has brought me more joy, happiness and freedom than I would have ever imagined.

---

80   Eisenstein, C., 2021.

After reading Charles Eisenstein's *Sacred Economics*, I downsized to living with my partner's parents. This allowed me to decrease my mortgage expenses to be able to pay for my son's college. It also allowed my partner's mom to retire early and help take care of her grandsons. Splitting the cost of living between the four of us in one house decreased the cost for each of us. Splitting the chores helps each of us save time and have more time to do the things we want to do. Downsizing to a smaller space keeps me from buying items I don't need and allows me to share most of what I own. I now share clothes, including jewelry, with my sister-in-law, and since then I have received more compliments than ever before.

I don't buy anything unless I use it or need it. When traveling, I buy no knickknacks, either for myself or others. I enter the shops and admire the craftsmanship of different items or artwork, feeling gratitude for their skill to create such beauty in the world, without the need to own it. I pay attention to the amount of trash I produce, and consider it a success when I can skip the weekly waste collections. I give away or sell things I no longer need or repurpose them. I share my possessions with others. I decline free promotional items such as pens, balls, frisbees and cups. I buy used things, and I don't buy new ones before I use up the old. All of this has enriched my life and given me a new sense of purpose.

Bottled Water

Many people, mistrustful of public water because of our increasing awareness of contaminants, choose, ironically, to substitute it with bottled water. However, bottled water is also susceptible to contamination, as it often undergoes less stringent public health and environmental regulations compared to tap water. Water in plastic bottles has become more popular in recent years making it the fastest growing food industry worldwide. Sales are expected to double to $500 billion worldwide this decade.[81] As a result, plastic bottles are now a major problem.

---

[81] Bouhlel & Smakhtin, 2023.

These bottles and caps leach microplastics into the water they contain. A recent study analyzed 259 bottles of eleven globally sourced bottled water brands, purchased from 19 locations across nine different countries. The findings revealed a concerning reality – 93% of the bottles contained microplastic particles, with an average of 10.4 particles per liter. Alarmingly, this microplastic contamination level was nearly double that typically found in tap water.[82]

To prevent ourselves being contaminated by tiny particles of plastic, micro and nano plastics, we have to reduce our consumption of bottled water. This is especially important in places where clean, safe tap water is already provided. In the US, to meet the demand each year for bottled water, 17 million barrels of oil are required to produce the plastic. The impact made by bottled water on natural resources is 3,500 times greater than that made by tap water.[83]

Major corporations make billions of dollars off the water they pump out for little to no cost, damaging local ecosystems and impoverishing the lives of their residents.

In major US cities, Detroit, Phoenix, and Denver among others, big corporations are exploiting the municipality's water supply. Meanwhile, the inhabitants face financial hardships and water shortages. Unable to afford their water bill, many are forced to buy bottled water that comes from the same source that feeds their taps.[84] However this water can be between 240 and 10,000 times more expensive.[85]

The bottled water industry widens the global disparity between the billions of people who lack access to reliable water services and the others that enjoy water as a luxury. Figures for 2016 reveal that to provide safe drinking water worldwide would cost around $114 billion annually – less than half of the roughly $270 billion in global bottled water sales that year.[86]

---

[82] La Porta, E., et al. 2023. Microplastics and kidneys.
[83] Villanueva, C. M., et al. 2021. Health and environmental impacts of drinking water choices.
[84] Felton, R. 2023. Pepsi, Coke, and Nestlé top plastic violators list.
[85] Washington County. (n.d.). Bottled vs. tap water.
[86] Bouhlel & Smakhtin, 2023.

The escalating number of plastic bottles ending up as waste exacerbates the whole problem of plastic in the environment. In addition, large-scale water extraction for bottling can significantly lower groundwater levels. This in turn affects the availability of water for local communities, agriculture and natural ecosystems. Rivers, lakes and wetlands may run dry, leading to habitat loss for wildlife and damaging biodiversity. Furthermore, as a result of water bottling, the pollutants produced can concentrate in remaining water sources.

Water Filtration Systems

One wonderful alternative to bottled water is a water filtration system. There are many different filtration mechanisms to choose from. However, several factors need to be considered when picking which is right for you. Among the most effective systems are reverse osmosis, activated carbon and UV light. Certified bodies such as NSF International or the Water Quality Association (WQA) ensure that systems meet the required standard. You should also bear in mind the maintenance issues, including the frequency of filter changes and the ease of obtaining replacement parts. Evaluate both the initial cost and ongoing maintenance expenses. To lessen the environmental impact, choose biodegradable filters with longer lifespans; this will reduce the frequency of replacing them. Some manufacturers offer take-back programs for used filters.

Reverse Osmosis Filters

The reverse osmosis filter is the most effective at removing small particles like heavy metals, microplastic, pesticides, dissolved salts, chlorine, fluoride, even viruses and bacteria. However, this filter also removes beneficial minerals such as calcium, magnesium and potassium which are essential for health. Some advanced reverse osmosis systems remineralize the water after filtration, but with the remineralization canisters and water reservoir tanks, this system takes up more space than others. So you need to consider the amount of space you have available.

The thoroughness of reverse osmosis filtration means it takes longer and reduces the overall flow rate (gallons per minute of filtered water). This is one of the reasons why reverse osmosis filters are often used for drinking water only and are less suitable for other uses around the house such as bathing water. Another disadvantage is the high amount of water wastage (up to 4 gallons of wastewater per gallon of purified water).

Carbon Water Filtration Systems

If you suffer from chlorine sensitivity, or you are concerned about the absorption of substances through the skin, you might consider using carbon filters instead. These are preferable if your goal is to filter all water, not just drinking water. Carbon filters can filter more gallons per minute than reverse osmosis filters while maintaining adequate water pressure.

The activated carbon is made from a variety of carbon-rich materials such as coconut shells, coal, wood and peat. These natural materials do not decompose quickly. Also, coconut shells and wood are renewable resources, making them more environmentally friendly. Most carbon filters are still coated in a plastic casing and may add significant waste to landfills.

UV Water Filtration Systems

UV filtration systems are effective in disinfecting water by using ultraviolet light to kill or inactivate bacteria, viruses and other microorganisms present in the water. They are often added as the last step in other filtration systems.

The UV-C light used in these filtration systems penetrates the cell walls of microorganisms and damages their genetic material so they can't replicate or repair themselves. It's a chemical-free method and doesn't affect the taste or odor of water, but it's important to note that the water must be clear for UV to work well since cloudiness or sediment can block the light.

The UV-C light used in these filtration systems penetrates the cell walls of microorganisms and damages their genetic material so they can't replicate or repair themselves. It's a chemical-free method and doesn't affect the taste or odor of water, but it's important to note that the water must be clear for UV to work well since cloudiness or sediment can block the light.

Whichever filtration system you choose, it's very important to maintain it according to the manufacturer's instructions.

Don't Settle for Heavy Metal

Just as plastic accumulates in our bodies, so do heavy metals. They are called heavy because of their relatively high atomic weight and density in comparison with other metals. When they accumulate in the body they pose serious health risks, due to their toxicity and potential to cause harm to the body's organs and systems. Lead, arsenic, cadmium and mercury are the heavy metals that are most commonly associated with poisoning humans.[87]

Elevated levels of heavy metals in the body are significant contributors to various neurological disorders in both children and adults. This critical issue often remains under-recognized within our current healthcare system. Testing for them is tricky and requires specialist knowledge. As patients, we might spend thousands of dollars on diagnostic imaging, consulting different specialists, receiving different diagnoses and more prescription medications. We may end up being treated for different illnesses, not realizing that the real cause of our trouble is having elevated amounts of heavy metals in our bodies.

I have been through this myself. When a functional practitioner finally tested me for heavy metals, I was shocked that my mercury and lead levels were so high. When my partner got tested, his levels were even higher. We lived in a house built after 1978, with a carbon water filtration system and didn't eat much seafood. Where did all that heavy metal come from? Since heavy metals get stored in the bone, such high numbers wouldn't have shown up in my blood tests unless I was being continually exposed to

---

[87] Ewers, 2017.

them. The cause must have been something that I consumed regularly and in significant quantities. Could it be the pink Himalayan salt that I was so fond of using, not only on my avocados, but in all my cooking?

What about my favorite sea-salted dark chocolate?

To learn about potential exposures, watch the documentary *MisLEAD: America's Secret Epidemic* by Tamara Rubin, also known as multi-award-winning independent advocate for childhood lead poisoning prevention and consumer goods safety. Since July 2022, the work of Tamara Rubin also known as the Lead Safe Mama has been responsible for 5 product recalls (FDA and CPSC). To learn more about how much lead is in your salt and other products, visit: tamararubin.com

Just as plastic, broken down into micro and nano-plastic, is polluting our environment, so are heavy metals. Just because we can't see or taste them doesn't mean they're not there. Due to the interconnectedness of our global systems, what we consume and use at home is often linked to practices and consequences abroad, revealing a cycle of exposure that cannot be ignored. With the same indifference with which the U.S. military used the chemical herbicide Agent Orange as a weapon in the Vietnam War, we are dumping our trash and all its toxic consequences on Third World countries, from whom we then import foods and other products. If it's in their air, soil and food, then it gets into ours.

Another source of heavy metal poisoning is improperly coated food containers. Cookware, plates and hand-painted pottery all may leak heavy metals into our food. Lead-based paints, medicines (including herbal supplements), contaminated food like fish and other seafood including seaweed, are also possible sources.[88] Smoking cigarettes is a well-known risk that delivers many toxic substances into the body including cadmium, lead, arsenic and chromium. E-cigarettes have been shown to release lead and manganese (both associated with causing Parkinson's disease) from their metal coil that gets heated to vaporize the liquid.[89] Further studies

---

88   Ewers, 2017.
89   Holm Johansen, 2019.

reveal the presence of arsenic and lead in the liquid prior to contact with the metallic coil.[90] Metal tooth fillings, including silver and amalgam, are toxic; amalgam fillings contain mercury. Additionally, some alloys contain nickel, which can cause inflammation of the gums. It has been estimated that, in the US, half of all dentists are still using dental amalgam as a cheap option for filling teeth.[91]

Heavy metals are a root cause of common neurological disorders, gastrointestinal autoimmune diseases and disorders associated with increased oxidative stress and cellular dysfunction. Once present in the body, they are not easy to deal with as they become stored in the bone; blood tests will only reveal their presence if our exposure to these toxins is ongoing. As we age, our bone density changes and these accumulated heavy metals are released into our bloodstream, with many resulting health problems.

Provocation agents such as DMSA (Dimercaptosuccinic acid) are used to move these heavy metals out of the bone and into the bloodstream. Chelation, a form of therapy which uses chemical compounds that form strong bonds with metals, is then employed to pass them out from the body. Patients must have good health and nutrition before starting this process. If not, the sudden influx of heavy metals, released after years of accumulation in the tissues, can lead to toxicity that the body may not be able to adequately handle and expel.[92]

Natural Ways to Get Rid of Heavy Metals

There is a wide variety of foods that can help detoxify our bodies and act as natural chelating agents. Nutrient-dense options include wild blueberries, spirulina, chlorella, fresh cilantro and garlic, with garlic considered as effective as standard prescription drugs. Pectin-rich fruits and vegetables like pears, green apples, citrus fruits, cabbage, grapes, beets and carrots

---

90 Broadfoot, 2022.
91 Burhenne, 2021.
92 Ewers, 2017.

are also beneficial. For vegetarian sources of protein, bear in mind that carrots, whole grains, oatmeal, spinach, turnips, papayas, plums, grapes and pomegranates all contain necessary amino acids. Sulfur-rich foods such as onions, cauliflower, cabbage, broccoli and brussels sprouts can also aid in detoxification, along with foods containing alpha-lipoic acid like peas, broccoli, spinach and rice bran.[93]

The Takeaways:

- Detoxify your home.
- Wear natural materials whenever possible.
- Try to lower your plastic use and pay attention to the kind and amount of trash you produce.
- Carry a designated stainless-steel water bottle that can last you for years. Mine is 32 oz.
- Use separate stainless-steel cups for coffee, tea, and water to avoid mixing flavors.

---

[93] Denny, 2017.

Chapter 10

A Functional Approach to Health

> *Throughout your life, the most profound influences on your health, vitality, and function are not the doctors you have visited, surgery, or other therapies you have underwent. The most profound influences are the cumulative effects of the decisions you make about your diet and lifestyle on the expression of your genes.*
>
> Jeffrey Bland, Ph.D., FACN

Why Functional Medicine?

As we have seen, scientific medicine, medical technology, global capitalism, consumerism and the food industry have advanced together. To separate our medical system from the outside interests that have brought it into being is nearly impossible.

Based on Senate Office of Public Records data, calculated by OpenSecrets:

> *In 2021 alone, there were nearly 15,000 active lobbyists and totaled lobbying spending reached $3.77B.*[94]

It has been estimated that since the early 2000s, the amount spent by big companies on lobbying politicians has regularly exceeded the combined House-Senate's own budget.[95] Through their financial capability, big corporations have been able to influence both lawmakers and popular opinion alike.

Conventional medicine has been similarly influenced by those holding the purse strings, be they government, industry or private individuals. As a result, healthcare is now split up into so many different disciplines that it can't work properly. It may be excellent at providing emergency medicine,

---

94 Auble, Glavin, & Quist, 2022.
95 Drutman, 2015.

surgical interventions, managing traumatic injuries, finding cures and discovering pharmaceutical remedies, but it is poor in acknowledging the importance of health – such things as lifestyle, nutrition and individual life circumstances.

Disregarding this holistic approach to healing, and disregarding the individual, we have come to lack understanding of how to live healthily. In so many ways, by downplaying the importance of a healthy lifestyle (including food and nutrition), we have ignored the root causes of disease.

Because of the gap that has grown between our healthcare system and an increasingly sicker society, a new holistic approach to medicine and nutrition – **functional medicine** – has emerged. Prompted by my extensive personal experience of the healthcare system as it now exists, I have not only become a practitioner of functional medicine myself, but also coach other nurses who feel as I do. In this chapter, I hope to encourage a greater number of people to consider the many benefits functional medicine can bring us all.

What Is Functional Medicine?

The functional medicine model is an individualized, patient-centered, science-based approach that empowers patients and practitioners to work together to address the underlying cause of disease and promote optimal wellness. It requires a detailed understanding of each patient's genetic, biochemical, and lifestyle factors, and leverages that data to direct personalized treatment plans that improve patient outcomes. By addressing the root cause rather than symptoms, practitioners become oriented to identifying the complexity of the disease. They may find that one condition has many different reasons, and, likewise, one cause may result in many other conditions. As a result, functional medicine treatment

> targets each individual's specific manifestations of disease in each individual. (The Institute for Functional Medicine, 2023).

The term 'functional medicine' was created in 1991 by Dr. Jeffrey Bland. It was the beginning of a discipline that merged basic medical science with expertise in clinical medicine to address the growing problems associated with chronic disease. That same year, together with his wife Susan Bland, they established *The Institute for Functional Medicine*.

Their mission was to educate and provide clinical support for implementing

> a systems-biology approach to the prevention and management of chronic disease, utilizing appropriate tools, including nutrition, lifestyle, exercise, structural, cognitive, emotional, and pharmaceutical therapies to meet the individual needs of the patient.[96]

As functional medicine is gaining popularity for its wonderful results in helping to get people healthy and off medications, it poses a threat to those institutions that profit off the sick, and has become prey to misinformation. But it is important to note that many professionals trained in our present healthcare system, such as myself, believe in and have added our contributions to this growing movement.

Functional medicine is real evidence-based science, practiced by physicians who obtain additional training and certifications in the functional medicine model. These practitioners spend hour-long appointments with their patients, getting to know them and their detailed health histories. They don't focus on treating the symptoms of a particular disease; instead, they concentrate on treating the disease itself. Their goal is to learn from the symptoms and get to the root cause of the issue.

---

96 The Institute for Functional Medicine, 2023.

A FUNCTIONAL APPROACH TO HEALTH

This new approach represents a breakthrough, not for its novel concepts or discoveries, but for its comprehensive nature. It uses various methods and disciplines to address health issues. Rather than targeting one aspect of health, such as one symptom or one organ of the body, practitioners consider the body as a whole and **all** the factors that could influence its health and wellbeing.

Prompted by functional medicine practitioners and their attempts to educate the public about the importance of genetics as the root cause of many health ailments, I have tested myself for the MTHFR gene mutation. After all, it has been estimated that more than 50% of the population has it without knowing. Since a lot of my symptoms, like gastrointestinal issues, food sensitivities, skin hives, and inability to sleep through the night were confirmatory, the results came as no surprise. I have a 70% mutation (one from each parent) of the C677T gene responsible for methylation. Methylation is critical in numerous biological processes and is essential for normal cellular function, growth, and repair. Having a 70% mutation means I have a 70% reduction in MTHFR enzyme activity responsible for converting folate (vitamin B9) into its active form, methylfolate, which is essential for DNA repair, neurotransmitter production, and detoxification. Since methylation is key in liver detoxification, this mutation reduces my ability to clear toxins, heavy metals, and environmental pollutants, leading to increased oxidative stress and inflammation.

This has been a life-changing discovery for me. I now take methylfolate (active folate) supplements instead of regular folic acid, which my body cannot efficiently convert. In addition, an adequate intake of vitamin B12 (as methylcobalamin), vitamin B6, and choline or betaine found in foods like eggs and beets help me prevent many complications that I am at risk for as a result of this gene mutation.

Functional medicine is also known as restorative medicine, as it enables the body to heal itself, rather than concentrating on the symptoms of its disease. A functional practitioner focuses on all aspects of their patient's life – lifestyle, nutrition, environment and stress levels – to bring about a healing environment. This holistic approach can forestall surgery and other invasive procedures.

Our aim is not to separate ourselves from conventional medicine but to complement it. The mainstream medical approach, practiced by licensed healthcare professionals, uses evidence-based, scientifically-proven methods to diagnose and treat diseases, relying on pharmaceuticals, surgery and other established therapies. Naturopathic medicine is a system of healthcare that emphasizes natural remedies, holistic approaches and the body's inherent healing abilities to prevent and treat illness. Functional medicine encompasses **all** evidence-based knowledge, from scientific to naturopathic. It serves as a bridge over the growing gap between technological and scientific advancements in medicine and the declining health of our population.

It is unhindered by all the competing financial interests which have come to dominate current practices in healthcare. It returns to the essence of medicine, addressing the root cause of each person's illness. Their circumstances and their emotions are not ignored but acknowledged. The body is not regarded as an assembly of different parts, with problematic ones to be cut out; patients are viewed as a whole and cared for holistically.

Functional medicine and its mission have spread across many health professions, creating a more health-conscious population. This has been brought about through education and placing the responsibility to respond back into the hands of each of us. We should each own our health, which is why I'm writing this book.

Health ownership should no longer be left only to physicians or healthcare providers. As quoted at the beginning of this chapter:

> *The most profound influences are the cumulative effects of the decisions you make about your diet and lifestyle.*[97]

---

[97]   Jeffrey Bland, The Institute for Functional Medicine, 2023.

Functional Nutrition

> Functional nutrition is the answer to some of the problems in health and healthcare today. A modality that works to not just support, but educate the patient in what's going on in their body and how making uniquely targeted diet and lifestyle modifications will shift the terrain and help them to meet their goals.
>
> Andrea Nakayama

Functional nutrition is the foundation of functional medicine. It helps individuals manage chronic diseases and achieve optimal health through personalized diets. As more and more people learn about functional nutrition, the health of our population will improve. Rather than merely treating symptoms, this approach addresses the root cause of health problems by applying science and technology to nutrition. As we learn how good food can heal us, we see how important it is to choose carefully what we eat.

Once you discover the benefits of healthy eating, you'll never want to go back to old habits – free doughnuts won't tempt you! Once your system has been cleaned out, the unpleasant reaction you get after eating them will put off any previous doughnut lover. Your taste buds will have undergone a change as a result of clean eating. You'll discover that doughnuts don't taste the way you remember them.

Food Intolerances

There is no single way toward healthy eating. Now that auto-immunological disorders, allergies and food sensitivities are so common, what works for one person, another cannot tolerate. Sometimes, complex investigative work is needed. Green tea (especially the now popular Matcha tea), kimchee, sauerkraut, dark chocolate, cheese, tomatoes and ripe bananas are generally considered healthy. But when I ate any of the above, I suffered from acid reflux. It took me a while to identify these foods as my triggers and to realize my body does not tolerate histamine well. Once I eliminated all high-histamine foods from my diet for 100 days, I was able to heal. After a while, I was slowly able to reintroduce them into my diet in small doses, without suffering any of the previous side effects.

Acid Reflux

Acid reflux is a potent symptom which should never be patched up with antacids. The body is trying to communicate an imbalance that needs to be addressed; if it is ignored, it could turn into a severe chronic disease. Figuring out what foods are best suited for an individual, based on their lifestyle, activity level and symptoms or reactions to different foods is challenging. It may require guidance from an expert, like a nutritional coach. Without assistance, we may self-diagnose incorrectly.

When we live with specific symptoms for a long time, it's easy to become immune to them. We tolerate them to the point that we do not even notice how much they are affecting our life. Living with different symptoms becomes the norm. A friend of mine was complaining about her chronic cough. When we went on vacation together, I recognized that it could be a symptom of acid reflux.

We took some time to do the investigative work together. She was exposed to a lot of abrasive chemicals at her job, and had recently noticed her chronic allergies getting worse. It was to a point that she couldn't wear makeup anymore. Her eyes would water while getting puffy and red. I could tell she had chronic inflammation issues that were getting out of control. She was skeptical of the changes I proposed and her husband was not supportive, but she knew she couldn't continue her old ways. Her body wouldn't allow it.

Together we established a plan. We began with simple things; replacing some of the abrasive cleaning supplies that she was using, with her own products, made with natural ingredients. Upon further investigation, I learned that for years she had been coloring her hair with two chemical dyes, but had become concerned about losing an abnormal amount of hair in recent months. She was able to switch from using a permanent hair color that had to be applied regularly (because otherwise the contrast accentuated the greys) to a semi-permanent blond hue that uses natural ingredients and plant extracts. The way this new hue washes off evenly throughout the hair looks more natural, and she no longer needs to apply it as frequently. She has also switched her make-up, ditching the eyeliner that was causing her issues. She now uses natural-based products with a list of clearly stated ingredients. Finally, we cleaned up her diet using the Whole30 protocol. The results were remarkable: the cough and the allergies went away and she has lost a few pounds as a bonus.

By treating inflammatory symptoms as normal, not listening and responding to what our body is telling us, we are missing our opportunity to prevent severe chronic illness.

Health, Nutrition, and Nurse Coaches

Part of the new way forward in medicine is the importance now placed on coaches in the fields of health, nutrition, and nursing. We no longer rely on prescription drugs – more on changes to lifestyle. The internet, with its unlimited access to information, has helped passionate individuals to promote their healthy lifestyles and guide others. Certification can be obtained in many ways. The Functional Nutrition Alliance, founded by Andrea Nakayama, is one I recommend.[98] Their Full Body Systems curriculum is exceptional.

We must understand the role of coaches within the healthcare system. In her program, Andrea makes a point of explaining it. She likens it to a pyramid, in which patients are placed at the bottom, physicians at the top, with the coaches that graduate from her program in the middle, filling what

---

98   Fxnutrition.com (website address correct at time of going to press, 2024).

has been a substantial void.

Coaches are not physicians: they can't prescribe medicines. However, emerging evidence is showing that, besides prescription drugs, the different lifestyle choices we make have a bearing on our health and our world. This is where nutritional coaches can help.

Andrea stresses that we should not discriminate between different approaches to medicine. Her coaches aim to bridge the gap between the implementation of best medical practice and the needs of individual patients. Following a doctor's diagnosis, a coach explores the changes their patients require in diet and lifestyle.[99] By identifying these necessary changes, the coach's assistance to physicians, who are limited by time and resources, is very important. The case of my friend's cough is a perfect example of how to work within that gap.

Functional Dentistry

Functional dentistry is a holistic approach to oral health that:

1. Focuses on prevention and root causes of oral diseases
2. Manages the oral microbiome
3. Addresses sleep-breathing issues
4. Offers dietary advice
5. Uses minimal or non-toxic materials
6. Creates personalized care plans
7. Recognizes the mouth-body connection

It includes holistic, integrative, biological, and natural dentistry practices.[100]

Learning about functional dentistry was eye-opening for me. For years I had bought antiseptic mouthwash, as instructed by dentists and dental

---

99 Nakayama, 25.
100 Burhenne, 2018.

hygienists. I rinsed my mouth with it every day, but still dark plaque built up around the base of my teeth, which needed regular cleaning to remove. I brushed, flossed, rinsed, and yet new cavities still developed. Then, functional dentistry taught me that rinsing with such abrasive solutions causes a microbial imbalance in the mouth. The mouthwash was killing not only the harmful bacteria but also the good ones that protect the teeth. After I stopped using it, to my surprise, the dark plaque stopped building up as it had done. I also learned about the role of scraping and brushing the tongue in eliminating bad breath and learned which foods cause it. What a difference when I removed them from my diet!

Today's market is saturated with dental care products, heavily advertised and promoted. How can we know which information is accurate, or which dentist to trust? How can we know which products have been thoroughly tested and are safe to use in the face of misinformation, skewed scientific research, and false claims by giant corporations wanting to manipulate the market?

Toothpaste is no exception. Until recently, I didn't realize how many top-selling toothpastes are full of harsh, controversial ingredients – like triclosan, sodium lauryl sulphate (SLS), cocamidopropyl betaine, propylene glycol (PEG), artificial sweeteners, diethanolamine (DEA) and parabens. I have mentioned some of these in the previous chapter.

Be sure to thoroughly inspect the toothpaste ingredient list before buying. If you are dissatisfied, why not try making your own with all-natural ingredients, instead?

Here is a recipe made popular by Dr Keesha:

HOMEMADE TOOTHPASTE RECIPE[101]

Ingredients:

- ½ cup coconut oil
- 3 tablespoons baking soda.
- 1/4 teaspoon finely ground xylitol powder
- 20 drops of peppermint, fennel, clove or cinnamon essential oil
- 10 drops myrrh extract if desired

Instructions:

1. Soften the coconut oil.
2. Add other ingredients and mix well.
3. Transfer mixture to small glass jars and coal.

---

[101] Included by kind permission from Dr. Keesha.

Fluoride

One of the most controversial toothpaste ingredients is fluoride. Whether to use it or not has become a big question recently, and if so, how much? The issue has become so serious that some states are currently facing lawsuits concerning fluoride, both for and against.

Fluoride has been proven to protect against cavities, so it has been added to toothpaste as well as to most of our public drinking water. The problem is how much is too much, since fluoride is toxic in excess. It's the dose that makes the poison. The Centers for Disease Control and Prevention (CDC) has set a recommended level of 0.7 mg of fluoride per liter in drinking water to help prevent tooth decay and promote oral health.[102]

If you want to know how much fluoride is in your drinking water, and whether it is within the recommended value, you can contact your city municipality for information, or visit: epa.gov

If you use water filtration systems to filter out the fluoride that's in your drinking water, then perhaps using a toothpaste that contains fluoride is a good idea. If you are already consuming the recommended fluoride levels in your water, then opting out of fluoride in toothpaste might be better for you.

If you've spotted white streaks, spots, or patches on your children's teeth, as I have, it might be a sign of fluorosis (excessive fluoride intake). The fluoride level in the water supply needs to stay within the safe recommended levels, but what about individual differences in size, age, and daily amount of water consumed? An optimal level for a toddler is much different from that for an adult.

To lessen the amount of toxins entering my body, I checked for them in my food, cleaning supplies, and cosmetics. I was aware of toxins in makeup and shampoo. Since I have curly hair, their detrimental effect was

---

102 Huberman, 2024.

hard not to notice. I never thought to look into toothpaste, yet it turns out toothpaste is one of the top products needing inspection. I exchanged highly commercialized products for clean and simple ones like Hello and Boka. These use natural ingredients such as hydroxyapatite, the main mineral component of tooth enamel. I also brush my teeth with herbal products, such as Isha Life Herbal and Himalaya Botanique toothpaste, or I make my own. Since then the health of my teeth and my mouth overall has improved significantly. My teeth have become much less sensitive to acidic fruits and cold temperatures; also, the sloughing skin[103] inside my mouth has completely disappeared.

We should realize that brushing teeth after meals is abrasive, especially after eating fruit. It is best to brush before breakfast and to wait an hour or two after the day's last meal to brush before going to bed. If you are concerned about the color of your teeth, do not resort to abrasive whitening strips. Try Dr. Keesha's homemade tooth whitener along with her oil-pulling recipe. Oil pulling is an ancient practice rooted in Ayurvedic medicine, where oil is swished around in the mouth for some time to promote oral health and hygiene. It detoxifies the mouth, potentially whitening teeth, balancing oral pH, freshening breath and combating bacterial and viral organisms that can cause tooth decay and gum disease.

---

[103] Sloughing of the skin refers to the shedding or peeling off from the outer layer of the skin.

DR. KEESHA'S HOMEMADE TOOTH WHITENER[104]

Ingredients:

- 1/4 cup calcium carbonate powder
- 1-2 packets powdered stevia
- 1/4 cup MCT oil
- Essential oils of choice (peppermint, cinnamon or fennel)

Instructions:

1. Mix all ingredients in a high-powered blender until smooth.
2. Transferred to a glass jar.

---

104 Included by kind permission from Dr. Keesha.

OIL PULLING MIXTURE

Ingredients:

- 1 cup organic cold-pressed sesame oil
- 10 drops clove essential oil
- 10 drops cinnamon essential oil
- 10 drops peppermint essential oil

Instructions:

1. Mix the ingredients in a glass jar.
2. Use 1-2 teaspoons in your mouth each morning and swish for 20 minutes.
3. Spit used oil into an old supplement container, not in your sink as oil will clog your plumbing.
4. Finish by scraping your tongue and brushing and flossing your teeth.

Functional Orthodontics

It was following the extraction of my wisdom teeth, and those of my son, that I learned about functional orthodontics. Functional orthodontics is a holistic approach to orthodontic treatment that focuses on correcting the underlying causes of dental and jaw misalignments, rather than just straightening teeth. This method believes that many orthodontic issues stem from environmental factors and improper oral habits, rather than genetics alone. It aims to improve overall facial structure, jaw alignment, and breathing function, often starting treatment earlier than in traditional orthodontic practice. Functional orthodontics typically uses removable or fixed appliances to guide jaw growth and development, expand dental arches, and create proper space for teeth, without extractions or the use of surgery.

Expansion of the jaw in a noninvasive manner can be achieved through techniques like palatal expanders,[105] myofunctional therapy,[106] and orthodontic and functional appliances.[107] They are often employed while children and teenagers are still growing, and the jaw is still developing and thus more malleable.

There is an alternative and functional approach to nearly every aspect of our health. It is usually the least invasive, therefore preventing unwanted side effects. Be sure to research functional ways before consenting to invasive interventions, so that you won't regret your decisions. It may protect you from disappointing outcomes that you won't be able to reverse.

---

[105] These devices are commonly used in children to gradually widen the upper jaw (maxilla). They apply gentle pressure to the palate, encouraging the bones to separate and create more space.
[106] Exercises and techniques designed to improve oral muscle function can contribute to proper jaw growth and development.
[107] Some removable or fixed appliances can guide jaw growth and expand the arches to address overcrowding or bite issues.

Lifestyle Medicine

Lifestyle medicine is an evidence-based approach that uses lifestyle changes to prevent, treat, and reverse chronic diseases. Certified practitioners prescribe treatments such as plant-based diets, exercise, regular sleep, stress management, substance avoidance, and social engagement as primary treatment methods. As with functional medicine, this approach aims to reshape healthcare by improving results, reducing expenses, and enhancing patient experience. Lifestyle practitioners are often trained in functional medicine and vice versa. With functional medicine, the aim is to find the root cause of the patient's illness, making use of the disciplines of genetics and biochemistry. Lifestyle medicine focuses on working with patients to improve their daily decisions concerning their overall health. It can also eliminate the root causes of illness by coaching patients in how to change their unhealthy behaviors.

It's hard to explain the difference between functional and lifestyle medicine, but let me give examples of patients who might benefit from one more than the other. Someone with a diagnosed chronic disease, such as heart disease, stroke, diabetes, obesity, metabolic syndrome, chronic obstructive pulmonary disease, and certain types of cancer may benefit from a lifestyle medicine practitioner. It might well be that their condition has been caused by unhealthy habits, such as smoking, unhealthy eating, and physical inactivity. On the other hand, a patient who leads a healthy lifestyle but still presents with symptoms where the root cause is difficult to identify may benefit more from a functional medicine practitioner.

Functional Nursing

Considering the current challenges within our healthcare system and our society overall, it is not a surprise that burnout amongst healthcare professionals is at an all-time high. If you were to ask nurses for the reason behind their career choice, you would most likely hear, "I want to help people." But in reality, nursing can often feel nothing like being a help. In fact, it often feels more like hindering, hurting, inappropriate, frustrating, forceful, and disagreeable.

Circumstances such as these are a daily occurrence in the life of a practicing nurse:

1. A patient with type II diabetes, after a coronary artery bypass graft surgery, whom you just spent an hour educating about healthy eating, to whom you must now serve a hospital's clear liquid tray for breakfast, full of all the things that you listed as "should not be consumed," including sugar substitutes.
2. An intubated patient, whose death is inevitable, unable to make decisions, whose life is being prolonged with interventions that cause immense pain.
3. A verbally abusive patient, admitted for drug and alcohol overdose, who threw their breakfast milk carton across the room to get attention while you were caring for your other patient.
4. A homeless patient who has been stabilized and discharged back onto the streets in paper scrubs because their clothes, when admitted, got cut up in the emergency department.
5. The newly paralyzed patient, scared to be left alone, seeks constant attention that you cannot provide.

On other occasions, instead of feeling like I've helped my patients, I feel as if I've reinforced their disease-causing lifestyle by providing them with pharmaceuticals. We have done this so much that they now expect it. Is it helpful or hindering? Is it empowering, or does it just make them more dependent? There is an emphasis on critical thinking in the nursing profession – but how about an emphasis on functional thinking? Do the services we provide make patients more functional or dysfunctional?

Nursing, as the largest workforce in healthcare, holds immense potential to transform patient care. Nurses are not only skilled clinicians but also compassionate caregivers with the expertise and patient-centered approach needed to support meaningful lifestyle and dietary changes. However, their contributions are often confined to hospitals and clinics, limited by outdated protocols that restrict their ability to innovate and expand their roles.

It's time to empower nurses to explore new, holistic ways of caring for and nurturing patients beyond traditional healthcare systems. Nurses should play a central role in preventative care, bringing their passion, expertise, and creativity to the forefront. The world needs functional nursing—an approach emphasizing prevention, sustainability, and true healing.

For this shift to occur, systemic changes are essential. Governments must prioritize the well-being of the public over the interests of powerful corporations. They must confront the harm caused by health misinformation and the adverse effects of laws, regulations, and subsidies that undermine public health. This includes implementing new policies and guidelines to protect against the manipulation of food and nutrition, which are fundamental to health and healing.

Nurses can lead the change by providing data and evidence of their cost-saving and health-improving measures. These efforts can influence reforms in medical insurance and create pressure for systemic change. By leveraging their unique skills and advocating for meaningful reforms, nurses have the power to reshape the future of healthcare and bring about a more equitable, preventative, and patient-focused system.

It is challenging for nurses to see themselves as independent practitioners. We may feel incapable since we can't prescribe medications and we aren't physicians. Nursing schools don't help in building the confidence nurses need to flourish in their professions. Instead, we're made to feel imprisoned within a broken system.

Nursing nowadays is far removed from nurturing. We often feel we are causing more pain and suffering, rather than creating health and healing. Although we may feel discouraged, let's not be defeated. It is time we nurses reclaim what was once the original purpose of our profession.

Emily Nagoski, in her book, *Come as You Are*,108 refers to each individual's inner essence as a garden. We tend to our gardens based on what we learn and what we experience throughout our lives, with childhood being the most relevant. Some learn to tend to their gardens early in life and maintain the habit, which enables them to produce incredible fruits. Some forget much of what they once learned, but still manage. Others are never even shown the way to their gardens, let alone how to take care of them. As healthcare practitioners, let's start by providing 'gardening assistance', so that everyone's inner essence can bloom!

Can you imagine powerful nursing expertise applied outside of the hospital system? Can you imagine being coached by a skilled nurse, who not only has therapeutic communication skills but who supports your innate abilities – who encourages what is best for you? Can you imagine nurse mentorship services, set up to prevent burnout among healthcare practitioners? Can you imagine empowered patients who understand their bodies and can make the best decisions for themselves?

If you can imagine all this, then you know the impact functional medicine, including functional nursing, can have on our current system.

Nurse Coaching

Nurse coaching is the "how" behind functional nursing. The current requirements for becoming a nurse coach are a bachelor's degree in nursing science, at least five years of clinical practice, 60 CEUs (continuing education hours) in specific topics of relevance, and being supervised over the coaching of ten different clients, for a total of 60 hours. Following this, we are allowed to take the nurse coach certification exam! Passing the required examination qualifies a nurse coach to work with individual clients in their private businesses, or hospitals.

---

108 Nagoski, E. (2021).

Nurse coaches empower and motivate through the following six-step process:

1. **assessment** – establishing relationship and identifying readiness for change
2. **diagnosis** identifying opportunities, issues and concerns
3. **outcome** identification establishing person-centered goals
4. **planning** creating the structure of the coaching interaction
5. **implementation** empowering and motivating the individual to reach goals
6. **evaluation** assisting the individual to determine the extent to which goals are achieved[109]

Hiring nurse coaches in hospital settings promises good results. Caring for our caregivers, so that the caregivers can continue to care for our patients, is fundamental to alleviating the current healthcare crisis. As previously mentioned in Chapter 2, the shortage of caregivers is affecting the safety of our patients. All hospitals should address this as their top priority.

Some hospitals are already doing so and are hiring nurse coaches to help overcome these problems. The results are incredible. Through listening to and acknowledging the staff, small changes with big consequences are being made. Improved retention rates mean improved quality of care, increased job satisfaction, and increasing patient satisfaction scores. Providing one-on-one coaching assistance to new or experienced or burnt-out staff makes all the difference!

In their private practice, using the six-step nursing process, nurse coaches are able to tailor their knowledge and clinical experience to individual clients' needs and life situations. The great advantage in providing care this way is that the clients are the ones establishing goals for themselves; it is not the practitioner who tells them what to do. The nurse coach is there to assist.

---

[109] Southard, 2020.

A FUNCTIONAL APPROACH TO HEALTH

For example, different clients with type II diabetes may have different goals. One may want to change their diet and lifestyle to not need medications, while another may want to learn to control their blood sugar better while being on medications and taking insulin. Yet another might have been hospitalized for ketoacidosis[110] in the past and wants to learn preventative measures. The same principles of the six-step nursing process are applied in coaching clients with other diseases or coaching healthy individuals who would like some assistance in reaching their goals. Nurse coaches can work with the client's family and their team of physicians, if needed.

Nurse coaches could be employed by insurance companies to reduce their costs. This signals new possibilities in healthcare, as currently, most insurance companies do not cover the cost of a functional doctor, nurse, or coach. Ironically, some are beginning to employ nurse coaches but not covering the cost of their services. Instead, patients are often forced to foot the bill themselves or use a health savings account. Because of this, the benefits of preventing or managing chronic lifestyle diseases are often inaccessible or limited among the very people who may need them most.

There is something fundamentally wrong here. Insurance companies should be spearheading change, instead of creating barriers to the improvement of our society's overall health. Their refusal to cover medical services provided by highly trained physicians, who specialize in addressing the underlying causes of chronic diseases, is mind-boggling, considering how this would significantly reduce healthcare costs.

I hope that insurance companies will make a greater effort to involve functional nurses and nurse coaches, making such interventions a priority or even a requirement.

---

[110] Ketoacidosis is a serious medical condition that can occur in individuals with diabetes, particularly those with type 1 diabetes. Dangerously high levels of ketones are produced in the blood when the body breaks down fat instead of glucose for energy.

Holistic Care

The part can never be well unless the whole is well.

Socrates

Holistic medicine, holistic healing, holistic care, and holistic nursing are not new ideas. Some of these concepts date back to the earliest days of human civilization. We have had the wisdom to recognize their importance since our very beginning. The idea of healing the whole person, rather than focusing on specific illnesses, body parts, or symptoms, has always been well known. Why is it that now we are struggling to incorporate it into our practice?

After discovering that germs were the cause of diseases, Western medicine shifted its focus to intervention. Diseases were treated as invaders, with drugs like penicillin as the weapon of choice. This approach neglected lifestyle, environment, and emotional factors in treating health disorders. The emphasis was on treating symptoms rather than promoting overall wellness. Patients became passive, expecting medicine to 'fix' them.

Over time, the limitations of this approach emerged. Some treatments proved harmful, and many chronic conditions resisted purely medical solutions. This realization took nearly a century to develop.

How did we miss the big picture? Some of it is due to the reasons stated above and described throughout this book. But perhaps the state of the world that we see about us reflects our inner state as individuals. If that is the case, then we all have work to do. If society is fractured and fragmented, so are the systems within which we function. If the medical, educational, and political systems are fractured, so is our planet. We cannot fix the systems without first fixing ourselves. If we continue to pretend that there is nothing wrong with the way we live, we will self-destruct.

It must start with the self. As we are taught as nurses:

> *Self-development is accepting personal responsibility for one's learning and development that involves self-reflection, self-assessment, self-evaluation, and self-care.* [111]

We may have the greatest intentions of helping others and healing the entire world, but if we lack self-awareness, our actions will fail to have the effect that we desire. We should be conscious of our motives; what drives the actions we choose to take?

With the advantages of having comfortable lives, not having to worry too much about food and shelter, the power to respond to our current situation lies in our hands. We have the means that many others do not. In expressing our gratitude for this, we must now take action – stop exploiting others and start saving precious resources for future generations.

Although changes must happen at the legislative level, this journey begins with self-care. We should all start engaging in health-promoting behaviors, feelings, and attitudes – adopt a healthier lifestyle – enhance inner balance and well-being. We should explore the emotional, social, and spiritual domains of our existence.

Throughout human history, the yearning to simplify the way we live has been a constant. We have developed tools to help us live more comfortably. Now that we have achieved this, more than any previous generations, we are poisoning ourselves and our planet to the point of self-endangerment. It is not only viruses and diseases that we need to fear, but also our collective actions and their profound impact on the rest of our world.

Let us then, through self-awareness and with minds focused on compassion, make thoughtful choices. Through meaningful actions and choices, let us

---

111 Southard et al., 2020.

shift our disease-oriented healthcare system toward self-care, improving the health of ourselves and our planet.

Appendix I Resources

Want to take the next step? Visit functionalnursing.com to learn more about Functional Nursing and explore the coaching packages designed to support your healing journey.

Part I: The Healthcare Crisis

After Tristan's death, her father Ron Smith, along with her sisters and the rest of the family, became activists for change and nursing advocacy, facilitating and supporting many campaigns. Please support their efforts by following Ron Smith's Facebook.

To sign up for the latest updates and to get involved with nursing advocacy campaigns visit: nursingworld.org

Part II: Reclaiming Health

CHAPTER 4: THROUGH MINDFULNESS TO AWARENESS

Tools to practice mindfulness and develop awareness.

- For the Isha Institute of Inner Science, and Inner Engineering Program, visit: isha.sadhguru.org
- To cultivate a new personality and create a new personal reality, visit: drjoedispenza.com

To learn more about misinformation and the impact of social media, watch:

- Jeff Orlowski's *The Social Dilemma* documentary (2020).

CHAPTER 5: CREATING HEALTH INSIDE AND OUT

For guidance in meditation practices, visit:

- isha.sadhguru.org
- drjoedispenza.com

CHAPTER 6: LISTENING TO THE BODY'S NEEDS.

- To become an "Earth Body" visit: consciousplanet.org and join the "Save Soil" movement.
- For The Functional Nutrition Lab and to become an empowered expert in your own health, or to sign up for a year-long "Full Body Systems" training with Andrea Nakayama, visit: andreanakayama.com or fxnutrition.com
- To learn more about Dr. Wahls protocol and her amazing work on managing multiple sclerosis and autoimmune disorders, visit: terrywahls.com
- How to Understand and Use the Nutrition Fact Label – visit: fda.gov

Here is the link: https://www.fda.gov/food/nutrition-facts-label/how-understand-and-use-nutrition-facts-label

For additional information on how not to get tricked by misleading advertisement claims on products, visit healthline.com

Misleading Food Labels to Watch For

- **Light**: Light products often have reduced calories or fat, but they may achieve this by adding fillers, thickeners, or artificial flavors. Always check if these additives affect the overall nutritional value.
- **Multigrain**: "Multigrain" implies a variety of grains, but it doesn't guarantee any health benefit. For a healthier choice, look for products labeled "100% whole grain" or "whole grain first ingredient."

- **Natural**: The term "natural" is not well-regulated. It doesn't mean the absence of artificial flavors, colors, or preservatives. Always scrutinize the ingredients list.
- **Organic**: While organic products avoid synthetic pesticides and fertilizers, organic snacks, desserts, or processed foods can still be high in calories, sugar, and unhealthy fats.
- **No Added Sugar**: This label only means that no extra sugar was included during processing. Products like fruit juices may still be high in naturally occurring sugars. Always consider the total sugar content.
- **Low-Calorie**: Some low-calorie products reduce calories by shrinking portion sizes, using artificial sweeteners, or omitting nutrients like fiber or protein that contribute to satiety.
- **Low-Fat**: Removing fat often involves compensating with sugar, salt, or artificial flavorings. These changes can make the product less satisfying and potentially more harmful.
- **Low-Carb**: Many low-carb products are still heavily processed and may rely on artificial ingredients or unhealthy fats to improve texture or flavor.
- **Made With Whole Grains**: Look for terms like "whole wheat" or "whole oats" high in the ingredient list. Be cautious with products using vague claims like "contains whole grains."
- **Fortified or Enriched**: Adding nutrients doesn't necessarily make up for unhealthy elements like excessive sugar, sodium, or unhealthy fats.
- **Gluten-Free**: Gluten-free diets are essential for individuals with celiac disease or gluten sensitivity but aren't inherently healthier. Many gluten-free products are made with refined starches that lack nutrients.
- **Fruit-Flavored**: Always verify if real fruit is used. Products may include fruit concentrates or artificial flavors instead of actual fruit.
- **Zero Trans Fat**: Look for "partially hydrogenated oils" in the ingredient list, as these are the primary sources of trans fat even in "zero trans fat" products.

Hidden Sources of Sugar

Be aware of various hidden names for sugar in ingredient lists:

- **Types of Sugar**: Examples include beet sugar, brown sugar, coconut sugar, cane sugar, raw sugar, demerara sugar, turbinado sugar, muscovado sugar, evaporated cane juice, panela, and confectioner's sugar.
- **Types of Syrup**: Watch for syrups like tapioca syrup, sorghum syrup, malted barley syrup, corn syrup solids, high-fructose corn syrup, agave nectar, malt syrup, maple syrup, and rice syrup.
- **Other Added Sugars**: Sugars may also appear as molasses, barley malt, lactose, fruit juice concentrate, maltodextrin, crystalline fructose, sucrose, glucose solids, mannose, or diastatic malt powder.

Additionally:

- **Serving Sizes**: Always check the serving size on packaging, as misleadingly small portions can hide the true impact of certain ingredients.
- **Ingredient Order**: Ingredients are listed by weight. If sugar or refined grains appear near the top, the product is likely less healthy.
- **Claims vs. Facts**: Marketing claims on the front of packaging are often designed to be enticing. Rely on the nutrition facts panel and ingredient list for the full picture.

Whole30

To learn the details of the **Whole30 Program,** visit: whole30.com

Wahls Paleo Plus

To learn more about a healthy ketogenic diet such as Wahls Paleo Plus and Dr. Terry Wahls' research-backed strategies for managing multiple sclerosis and other autoimmune diseases, visit: terrywahls.com

Lectins

To learn more about lectins and the hidden dangers in "healthy" foods that cause disease and weight gain, as well as purchase quality products and supplements, visit: gundrymd.com

Magic of Cooking

For healthy recipes that work with different diets and protocols, visit: downshiftology.com

CHAPTER 7: HOLISTIC EATING

Composting

- To learn more about composting and how to start, visit: epa.gov

Here is the link: https://www.epa.gov/recycle/composting-home#worms

- If you don't have a space for composting, consider participating in a local municipal or community composting program that may collect your food scraps or offer a designated location where you can drop them off. Visit:

https://www.epa.gov/sustainable-management-food/community-composting

or

wastenotcompost.com

- To purchase an electric composter, visit: mill.com

To hear *Nature is Speaking* by Conservation International, visit: conservation.org

CHAPTER 8: FROM HEALTHCARE TO SELF-CARE

- For the Ann Wigmore Natural Health Institute, and to learn more about the "Living Foods Lifestyle" program that teaches optimal health through chlorophyll-rich and cultured foods, visit: annwigmore.org
- To learn more about Vipassana meditation and the 10-day silent retreat, visit: dhamma.org
- For psychological, spiritual, and practical guidance in navigating life's most challenging situations, explore a blend of Japanese psychology methods such as Morita and Naikan, as well as the Kaizen philosophy. Visit: www.thirtythousanddays.org

CHAPTER 9 ELIMINATING TOXINS

Harmful Substances in Cosmetics

Simplified shoppers guide to avoid the dirty dozen found in cosmetics:

https://davidsuzuki.org/wp-content/uploads/2017/10/sustainable-shoppers-guide-dirty-dozen-cosmetics-ingredients.pdf

To learn about sustainable living, using natural ingredients, and how to take action to protect the environment, visit: davidsuzuki.org

Homemade Natural Substitutes

For more DIY recipes from Dr. Keesha who is an integrative medicine expert, visit: drkeesha.com

Essential Oils

For more DIY recipes using natural ingredients and essential oils, visit: aromatics.com

To learn more about essential oils and their healing properties, including more recipes and remedies, visit: naturallivingfamily.com

Gardening

For those seeking inspiration in the art of gardening and farming, watch:

The Biggest Little Farm (2019)

The Biggest Little Farm: The Return (2022) directed by John Chester.

Don't Settle for Heavy Metal

To learn more about Tamara Rubin's work and how much lead is in your salt and other products, visit: tamararubin.com

Here is the link:

https://tamararubin.com/2023/12/to-get-a-beneficial-amount-of-the-trace-minerals-found-in-some-salts-i-e-himalayan-celtic-real-salt-etc-you-would-need-to-eat-a-lethal-amount-of-salt/

- Watch Tamara's documentary "MisLEAD: America's Secret Epidemic-Fine Cut
- Watch the documentary "Intoxicated -While Mercury Rises" at intoxicated.vhx.tv
- To learn more about Sacred Economics and the works of Charles Eisenstein, visit: charleseisenstein.org

CHAPTER 10: A FUNCTIONAL APPROACH TO HEALTH

- For The Institute for Functional Medicine, visit: ifm.org
- To test for MTHFR, and other genetic mutations, as well as other functional tests, visit: mybodyfabulous.co.uk
- For wise traditions in food, farming, and the healing arts, visit: westonaprice.org

- Founded by a Cleveland dentist, Dr. Weston A. Price (1870-1948).
- To check the fluoride levels in your drinking water and get your tap water tested, visit: epa.gov
- Here is a link:

https://www.epa.gov/ground-water-and-drinking-water/local-drinking-water-information

- To find a Functional Dentist or for more information on how to prevent and reverse cavities and gum disease, or for more DIY toothpaste, mouthwash, and whitening pastes recipes, visit: Dr. Mark Burhenne, DDS at aksthedentist.com
- For the American College of Lifestyle Medicine, visit: lifestylemedicine.org

To work with me and learn more about functional nursing and nurse coaching, visit: functionalnursing.com, or email me at: kasiaosuch@functionalnursing.com

- NursePreneurs is a mentorship program that empowers nurses to monetize their knowledge, develop business skills, and help healthcare delivery evolve. To learn more, visit: nursepreneurs.com
- National Nurses in Business Association (NNBA) is the premier nursing organization for nurse entrepreneurs and a springboard for nurses transitioning from employees to entrepreneurs and business owners. To learn more, visit: nursesbusiness.com
- American Holistic Nurses Association (AACN) aims to illuminate holism in nursing practice, community, advocacy, research, and education. To learn more, visit: ahna.org

HEALTHCARE REVAMPED

Additional Functional, Holistic, and Restorative Medicine Practitioners

Dr. Anthony Youn is a board-certified plastic surgeon known as America's Holistic Plastic Surgeon. To learn more, visit: dryoun.com

Dr. Keesha Ewers is a board-certified Functional and Ayurvedic medical practitioner, as well as Doctor of Sexology and family practice ARNP (Advanced Registered Nurse Practitioner). To learn more, visit: drkeesha.com

David Permutter is a renowned neurologist whose expertise includes gluten issues, brain health and nutrition, and preventing neurodegenerative disorders. To learn more, visit: drperlmutter.com

Dr. Blake Livingood is a Doctor of Natural Medicine and the creator of The Livingood Daily Lifestyle. To learn more, visit: drlivingood.com

Dr. Dan Kalish is the founder of the Kalish Institute for Functional Medicine. To learn more visit: kalishinstitute.com

To learn more about a holistic approach to skincare and natural beauty, visit: peachesskincare.com

Appendix II References

- AABC (n.d.) *Highlights of 4 Decades of Developing the Birth Center Concept in the U.S.* American Association Of Birth Centers. https://www.birthcenters.org/history

- Abalo-Lojo, J. M., Paredes, D., & Domínguez, M. (2023). Olfactory training and aromatherapy in post-viral olfactory dysfunction: A systematic review. *Frontiers in Neuroscience, 17*, Article 10102705. https://doi.org/10.3389/fnins.2023.10102705

- Aly Sterling Philanthropy (2023) *Corporate Philanthropy: The Complete Guide for Businesses.* The Giving Institute. https://alysterling.com/corporate-philanthropy-guide/

- Ann Wigmore Natural Institute (n.d.) *Now Is The Time To Take Charge of Your Health: Ann Wigmore Natural Health, Beachfront Wellness Retreat.* Ann Wigmore Natural Institute. https://annwigmore.org

- Armstrong, K. (2019, September 25). *Interoception: How we understand our body's inner sensations.* Association for Psychological Science APS. https://www.psychologicalscience.org/observer/interoception-how-we-understand-our-bodys-inner-sensations

- Balwierz, R., Biernat, P., Jasińska-Balwierz, A., Siodłak, D., Kusakiewicz-Dawid, A., Kurek-Górecka, A., Olczyk, P., & Ochędzan-Siodłak, W. (2023). Potential Carcinogens in Makeup Cosmetics. *International Journal of Environmental Research and Public Health, 20*(6), 4780. https://doi.org/10.3390/ijerph20064780

- Bouhlel, Z., & Smakhtin, V. (2023, April 4). *How the bottled water industry is masking the global water crisis.* United Nations University. https://unu.edu/article/how-bottled-water-industry-masking-global-water-crisis

- Bowden, J., & Sinatra, S. (2015). *The great cholesterol myth: Why lowering your cholesterol won't prevent heart diseaseand the statin-free plan that will.* Fair Winds Press.

- Broadfoot, M. (2022, February). *E-cigarettes expose users to toxic metals such as arsenic, lead*. National Institute of Environmental Health Sciences. https://factor.niehs.nih.gov/2022/2/feature/3-feature-e-cigarettes-and-toxic-metals#:~:text=Through%20the%20EMIT%20study%2C%20Rule's,contact%20with%20the%20metallic%20coil

- Brown, E.R. (2017). *Rockefeller Medicine Men: Medicine and Capitalism in America*. Andesite Press.

- Burhenne, M. (2018, October 26). *Functional dentistry: Everything you need to know*. Ask the Dentist. https://askthedentist.com/functional-dentistry/

- Burhenne, M. (2021, October 26). *Mercury fillings dangers, who is at risk & removal checklist*. Ask the Dentist. https://askthedentist.com/mercury-fillings-safe/

- The Guardian. (2021, April 27). *California's biggest water user will have to stop draining the state dry, officials say*. Retrieved July 12, 2024, from https://www.theguardian.com/us-news/2021/apr/27/california-nestle-water-san-bernardino-forest-drought

- Casey, L. (2021). *Lifestyle medicine defined*. American College of Lifestyle Medicine | Redesigning Healthcare, Better. https://lifestylemedicine.org/What-is-Lifestyle-Medicine

- Cechin-De La Rosa, C., Holm Johansen, S., Mettler, D. (Writer), & Holm Johansen, S. (Director). (2019, November 17). *Big Vape (Episode 2)*. [TV series episode]. In C. Collins, L. Tenaglia, & J. Caterini (Executive Producers), Broken, Netflix.

- Center for Biological Diversity. (n.d.). *Ocean plastics pollution*. Center for Biological Diversity. https://www.biologicaldiversity.org/campaigns/ocean_plastics/

- Cohen, P. (2020, June 24). *Roundup Maker to Pay $10 Billion to Settle Cancer Suits*. The New York Times. https://www.nytimes.com/2020/06/24/business/roundup-settlement-lawsuits.html

REFERENCES

- Center of Disease Control and Prevention (2020) Community Water Fluoridation. Center for Disease Control and Prevention. https://www.cdc.gov/fluoridation/faqs/community-water-fluoridation.html#:~:text=Many%20communities%20adjust%20the%20fluoride,often%20called%20the%20optimal%20level).

- Center of Disease Control and Prevention (2022) What is Epigenetics? Center for Disease Control and Prevention. https://www.cdc.gov/genomics/disease/epigenetics.htm

- Cimmino I, Fiory F, Perruolo G, Miele C, Beguinot F, Formisano P, Oriente F. Potential Mechanisms of Bisphenol A (BPA) Contributing to Human Disease. Int J Mol Sci. 2020 Aug 11;21(16):5761. doi: 10.3390/ijms21165761. PMID: 32796699; PMCID: PMC7460848.

- Corbley, A. (2022, May 9). American Produce has Lost As Much As 80% of Its Nutrition Since the 1950s. World at Large. https://www.worldatlarge.news/coffee-break-reads/2022/5/9/american-produce-has-lost-as-much-as-80-of-its-nutrition-since-the-1950s

- Danny, L. (2013, February 21). 7 Foods for Heavy Metal Detoxification. SF Spine Pain Relief Center. https://sfchiro.org/7-foods-for-heavy-metal-detoxification/

- Dispenza, J. (2014). You are the placebo: Making your mind matter. Hay House.

- Downs, C.A., Kramarsky-Winter, E., Fauth, J.E. et al. Toxicological effects of the sunscreen UV filter, benzophenone-2, on planulae and in vitro cells of the coral, Stylophora pistillata. Ecotoxicology 23, 175–191 (2014). https://doi.org/10.1007/s10646-013-1161-y

- https://link.springer.com/article/10.1007/s10646-013-1161-y

- Drutman, L. (2015, April 20). How Corporate Lobbyists Conquered American Democracy. The Atlantic. https://www.theatlantic.com/business/archive/2015/04/how-corporate-lobbyists-conquered-american-democracy/390822/

- *Eisenstein, C. (2021). Sacred Economics: Money, Gift, and Society in the Age of Transition. North Atlantic Books.*

- *The Guardian. (2021, August 5). Environmental impact of bottled water up to 3,500 times greater than tap water, study finds.* https://www.theguardian.com/environment/2021/aug/05/environmental-impact-of-bottled-water-up-to-3500-times-greater-than-tap-water

- *Ewers, K. (2017). Solving the autoimmune puzzle: The woman's guide to reclaiming emotional freedom and vibrant health.*

- *Ewers, K. (n.d.). DIY Autoimmune Home Detox. Dr. Keesha Healing from the Inside Out.* https://drsummits.s3.us-west-1.amazonaws.com/2021+Summits/Reverse+Autoimmune+Detox+Summit+4.0/Bonuses/Home-Detox-eBook.pdf

- *Faron, R. (2022, August 30). Microplastic in Blood Spotlight Health Emergency from Plastic Pollution. Discovery.* https://www.discovery.com/science/microplastics-in-the-blood

- *Felton, R. (2023, April). Pepsi, Coke, Nestlé top list of plastic violators in global cleanups, report finds. The Guardian.* https://amp.theguardian.com/us-news/2023/apr/23/pepsi-coke-bottled-water-consumer-reports

- *Gundry, S. R. (2017). The plant paradox: The hidden dangers in "healthy" foods that cause disease and weight gain. HarperCollins.*

- *Halden, R. U., Lindeman, A. E., Aiello, A. E., Andrews, D., Arnold, W. A., Fair, P., Fuoco, R. E., Geer, L. A., Johnson, P. I., Lohmann, R., McNeill, K., Sacks, V. P., Schettler, T., Weber, R., Zoeller, R. T., & Blum, A. (2017, June 20). The Florence Statement on Triclosan and Triclocarban. Environmental Health Perspectives, 125(6), 064501.* https://doi.org/10.1289/EHP1788

- *Holm Johansen, S. (Director). (2019, November 17). Big Vape [Television series episode]. Cechin-De La Rosa, C. (Executive Producer), Broken. Netflix.*

REFERENCES

- Hopkins, M. (2013, February 21). *Monsanto: Why We Sue Farmers Who Save Seeds.* CropLife News. https://www.croplife.com/crop-inputs/seed-biotech/monsanto-why-we-sue-farmers-who-save-seeds/

- Howard, J. (2023, March 16). *US Maternal Death Rate Rose Sharply in 2021, CDC data Shows, and Experts Worry the Problem is Getting Worse.* CNN Health. https://www.cnn.com/2023/03/16/health/maternal-deaths-increasing-nchs/index.html

- Huberman, A. (Host). (2024, January 31). *Fluoride Benefits/Risks & Vagus Nerve Stimulation* (No. 15) [Audio podcast episode]. Huberman Lab. https://www.hubermanlab.com/episode/ama-15-fluoride-benefits-risks-vagus-nerve-stimulation

- Institute of Integrative Nutrition (2022, December 2) *What Is Functional Nutrition?* Institute for Integrative Nutrition blog. https://www.integrativenutrition.com/blog/what-is-functional-nutrition

- Isha Institute of Inner Sciences (n.d) *What is Inner Engineering?* Isha Foundation. https://innerengineering.sadhguru.org

- The Institute for Functional Medicine (2023) https://www.ifm.org/about/our-mission-vision-and-deib-commitment/

- Jofili Pediatrics (n.d) *Functional Medicine.* Jofili Pediatrics Integrative Medicine. https://www.jofilipediatrics.com/functional-medicine

- Kummer, F. (2022, May 5). *Only About 5% of Plastic Waste Gets Recycled in US, New Report Says.* Science X Network. https://phys.org/news/2022-05-plastic-recycled.amp

- Kurani, N., Ortaliza, J., & Wager, E. (2022, February 25). *How has U.S. spending on healthcare changed over time?* Peterson-KFF Health System Tracker. https://www.healthsystemtracker.org/chart-collection/u-s-spending-healthcare-changed-time/

- Lacal, I., & Ventura, R. (2018, September 28). *Epigenetic Inheritance: Concepts, Mechanisms and Perspectives.* Front Mol Neurosci, Volume 11. https://doi.org/10.3389%2Ffnmol.2018.00292

- *Leadership Now Project (n.d.) Corporate Political Influence 101. Leadership Now Project.* https://www.leadershipnowproject.org/corporate-political-influence-101#

- *La Porta, E., Exacoustos, O., Lugani, F., Angeletti, A., Chiarenza, D. S., Bigatti, C., Spinelli, S., Kajana, X., Garbarino, A., Bruschi, M., Candiano, G., Caridi, G., Mancianti, N., Calatroni, M., Verzola, D., Esposito, P., Viazzi, F., Verrina, E., & Ghiggeri, G. M. (2023). Microplastics and kidneys: An update on the evidence for deposition of plastic microparticles in human organs, tissues and fluids and renal toxicity concern. International Journal of Molecular Sciences, 24(18), Article 14391.* https://doi.org/10.3390/ijms241814391

- *Mar-Solis, L. M., Soto-Dominguez, A., Rodriguez-Tovar, L. E., Rodriguez-Rocha, H., Garcia-Garcia, A., Aguirre-Arzola, V. E., Zamora-Avila, D. E., Garza-Arredondo, A. J., Castillo-Velazquez, U. (2021, October 20). Analysis of the Anti-Inflammatory Capacity of Bone Broth in a Murine Model of Ulcerative Colitis. National Library of Medicine. doi: 10.3390/medicina57111138*

- *Masley, S., & Bowden, J. (2016). Smart fat: Eat more fat. Lose more weight. Get healthy now. HarperCollins.*

- *Mazhari, M. (2019, September 5). What is functional orthodontics? Your Dental Health Resource: The Go-To Smile Guide.* https://yourdentalhealthresource.com/what-is-functional-orthodontics/

- *McDonald, J. (2023, February 17). Curbing America's Trash Production: Statistics and Solutions. Dumpsters.* https://www.dumpsters.com/blog/us-trash-production

- *Menigoz, W., Latz, T. T., Ely, R. A., Kamei, C., Melvin, G., & Sinatra, D. (2020). Integrative and lifestyle medicine strategies should include earthing (grounding): Review of research evidence and clinical observations. EXPLORE, 16(3), 152-160.* https://doi.org/10.1016/j.explore.2019.10.005

- *Modest, A. M., Prater, L. C., Naima, J.T. (2022, October). Pregnancy-Associated Homicide and Suicide: An Analysis of the National Vi-*

REFERENCES

olent Death Reporting System, 2008-2019. *Obstetrics & Gynecology*, 140(4), 565-573. doi: 10.1097/AOG.0000000000004932

- Montano L, Pironti C, Pinto G, Ricciardi M, Buono A, Brogna C, Venier M, Piscopo M, Amoresano A, Motta O. Polychlorinated Biphenyls (PCBs) in the Environment: Occupational and Exposure Events, Effects on Human Health and Fertility. *Toxics*. 2022 Jul 1;10(7):365. doi: 10.3390/toxics10070365. PMID: 35878270; PMCID: PMC9323099.

- Nagoski, E. (2021). *Come as You Are: Revised and Updated: The Surprising New Science That Will Transform Your Sex Life*. Simon & Schuster.

- Nakayama A.(2018, January) *Field Guide to Functional Nutrition: Your Passport to Navigating the New Healthcare Paradigm*. E-book, Functional Nutrition Alliance.

- National Geographic. (2021). *Welcome to Earth* [TV series]. Disney+.

- National Institute of Environmental Health Sciences. (n.d.). Bisphenol A (BPA). https://www.niehs.nih.gov/health/topics/agents/sya-bpa

- Natural Healers (n.d) *A History of Holistic Health*. Natural Healers blog. https://www.naturalhealers.com/blog/holistic-health-history/

- Newman, T. (2017, September 7). *Is The Placebo Effect Real?* Medical News Today. https://www.medicalnewstoday.com/articles/306437

- O'Neill Hayes, T., & Kerska, K. (2021, November 3). *Primer: Agriculture Subsidies and Their Influence on the Composition of U.S. Food Supply and Consumption*. American Action Forum. https://www.americanactionforum.org/research/primer-agriculture-subsidies-and-their-influence-on-the-composition-of-u-s-food-supply-and-consumption/

- Osteopathic Center for Healing (2018, September 26) *How Functional and Conventional Medicine Differ*.Osteopathic Center for Healing: Physical Medicine & Rehabilitation Physicians. https://www.drneilspiegel.com/blog/how-functional-and-conventional-medicine-differ

- *Philpotts, R. (2023, March 16). Top 5 Health Benefits of Bone Broth. BBC Good Food.* https://www.bbcgoodfood.com/howto/guide/health-benefits-of-bone-broth/amp

- *Resource Recycling. (2024, February 14). Scrap plastic exports drop to new low. Resource Recycling.* https://resource-recycling.com/plastics/2024/02/14/scrap-plastic-exports-drop-to-new-low/#:~:text=In%202023%2C%20the%20largest%20export,portion%20in%202023%20at%2037%25.

- *Rivo, S. (Director). (2019, November 27). Makeup Mayhem [Television series episode]. Cechin-De La Rosa, C. (Executive Producer), Broken. Netflix.*

- *Rodas, S. (2023, February 15). Majority of N.J. Residents Want Plastic Bag Ban Tweaked or Overturned Completely Poll Says. NJ Advanced Media.* https://www.nj.com/news/2023/02/dont-change-a-thing-about-njs-plastic-bag-ban-40-of-residents-say-in-new-poll.html?outputType=amp

- *Sadhguru. (2016). Inner Engineering: A Yogi's Guide to Joy. Spiegel & Grau, New York.*

- *Sadhguru (2021). Karma: A Yogi's Guide to Crafting Your Destiny. New Delhi, Thomson Press India Ltd.*

- *Safe Cosmetics. (n.d.). Nitrosamines.* https://www.safecosmetics.org/chemicals/nitrosamines/#

- *Saini, V., Garber, J., Brownlee, S. (2022, February 10). Nonprofit Hospital CEO Compensation: How Much Is Enough? Health Affairs Forefront. doi:10.1377/forefront.20220208.925255*

- *Schmidt, A. (2021, February 20). Regenerative & sustainable: What is the difference? Producers' Stories.* https://producersmarket.com/blog/what-is-the-difference-between-regenerative-sustainable-agriculture/

- *Sinclair, D. A., & LaPlante, M. (2019). Why we age and why we don't have to. Atria Books.*

REFERENCES

- Skelly, C. L., Cassagnol, M., & Munakomi, S. (2022, February 9). *Adverse events StatPearls NCBI bookshelf.* National Center for Biotechnology Information. https://www.ncbi.nlm.nih.gov/books/NBK558963/#_NBK558963_pubdet_

- Southard, M. E., Dossey, B. M., Bark, L., & Guilno-Schaub, B. (2020). *The art and science of nurse coaching: The provider's guide to coaching scope and competencies* (2nd ed.).

- Thomas, A. (2022, March 26). *A History of Holistic Health: Learn How Holistic Health's History Shaped the Practice It Is Today.* Natural Healers. https://www.naturalhealers.com/blog/holistic-health-history/

- United Nations University. (2015, September 15). *World loses trillions of dollars worth of nature's benefits each year due to land degradation: 50 million migrants may be created in a decade.* ScienceDaily. Retrieved April 25, 2023 from www.sciencedaily.com/releases/2015/09/150915090404.htm

- U.S. Environmental Protection Agency. (2023, December 12). *Community composting.* https://www.epa.gov/sustainable-management-food/community-composting

- U.S. Environmental Protection Agency. (2023, December 18). *Composting at home.* https://www.epa.gov/recycle/composting-home

- U.S. Food and Drug Administration. (2022). *1,4-Dioxane in cosmetics: A manufacturing byproduct.* FDA. https://www.fda.gov/cosmetics/potential-contaminants-cosmetics/14-dioxane-cosmetics-manufacturing-byproduct

- Villanueva, C. M., Garfí, M., Milà, C., Olmos, S., Ferrer, I., & Tonne, C. (2021). Health and environmental impacts of drinking water choices in Barcelona, Spain: A modelling study. *Science of The Total Environment, 795*, Article 148884. https://doi.org/10.1016/j.scitotenv.2021.148884

- Vipassana Meditation. (n.d.). https://www.dhamma.org/en-US/index

- Wahls, T. (2020). *The Wahls Protocol: A Radical New Way to Treat All Chronic Autoimmune Conditions Using Paleo Principles.* Avery.

- Wallheimer, B. (2018, June 7). *How Corporations Use Charitable Giving to Wield Political Influence.* Chicago Booth Review. https://www.chicagobooth.edu/review/how-corporations-use-charitable-giving-wield-political-influence

- Wang Y, Qian H. *Phthalates and Their Impacts on Human Health.* Healthcare (Basel). 2021 May 18;9(5):603. doi: 10.3390/healthcare9050603. PMID: 34069956; PMCID: PMC8157593.

- Washington County. (n.d.). *Bottled vs. tap water.* https://www.washingtoncountyor.gov/hhs/documents/bottled-vs-tap-waterpdf/download?inline

- Watson, K. (2019, July 10). *Is it possible to make a safe and effective sunscreen from scratch?* In D. R. Wilson (Ed.), Healthline. https://www.healthline.com/health/is-it-possible-to-make-a-safe-and-effective-sunscreen-from-scratch

- Zielinski, E., & Zielinski, S. A. (2021). *The Essential Oils Apothecary: Advanced Strategies and Protocols for Chronic Disease and Conditions.* Rodale Books.

www.ingramcontent.com/pod-product-compliance
Lightning Source LLC
Chambersburg PA
CBHW060453030426
42337CB00015B/1566